# The Blo Pressure Miracle

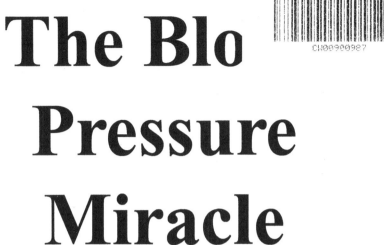

Frank Mangano

Strategic Book Publishing
New York, New York

Strategic Book Publishing
An imprint of Strategic Book Group
P.O. Box 333
Durham CT 06422
www.StrategicBookGroup.com

ISBN: 978-1-60911-087-1

Printed in the United States of America

# Medical Disclaimer

The information within this book is intended as reference material only, and not as medical or professional advice. Information contained herein is intended to give you the tools to make informed decisions about your lifestyle and health. It should not be used as a substitute for any treatment that has been prescribed or recommended by your doctor.

If you are currently taking medication for the treatment of high blood pressure (hypertension), continue to do so unless advised by your doctor to do otherwise. The author and publisher are not healthcare professionals, and expressly disclaim any responsibility for any adverse effects occurring as a result of the use of suggestions or information herein.

This book is offered as current information available about the management of hypertension, also known as high blood pressure, for your own education and enjoyment. If you have been told by a healthcare professional that you have high blood pressure, or if you have taken a blood pressure reading at a pharmacy or at home that is within the range of what is considered high, then it is imperative that you seek medical attention and the advice of your healthcare provider.

As always, never begin a dietary or exercise program without first consulting a qualified healthcare professional.

# Testimonials

Hi Frank,

I received your e-mail and would like to thank you for the valuable information in your book, "The Blood Pressure Miracle." Historically, my blood pressure has been 150/100 and most recently has increased to 170/120. Consistently following your suggested vitamin/herbal program and changing my overall lifestyle to include diet and exercise, my blood pressure is now 115/70! By successfully following your program, I was able to eliminate taking prescription medications with side effects. Thank you!

*D. Macur*
*Princeton, N.J.*

Frank,

I truly appreciate your help and even taking the time to talk with me about my blood pressure. I have been using your information and I am very happy to report GOOD NEWS! After just 6 weeks, my BP is already down in the 120's over 80's, and even as low as 70's.

I just wanted to say THANK YOU, and you can use this testimony on your site if you want. I know that the nutrition information has definitely helped.

GOD BLESS you and your efforts. I will recommend your book, if I run into people with BP, AND I usually do.

*Sincerely,*
*Mark G. Ross*

Hello Mr. Mangano:

I have been trying the techniques you offered in The Blood Pressure Miracle for one week now. My BP went from an average 130/95 down to 118/78 (today and yesterday's reading). That's BELOW NORMAL!!!!!!! This is amazing.

What triggered me to purchase the system was when my doctor prescribed a blood-pressure-lowering-medication. I stopped myself on the way to the pharmacy and decided to search on the Internet system for something more natural that didn't involve drugs. Your system seemed to be the best, so when I downloaded it and read the entire thing, I took notes and bought the proper groceries the following day and began my new lifestyle.

Thank you, Mr. Mangano, for knowledge that was so simple, which the nurses should have taught every single middle school student, let alone, my own FAMILY DOCTOR! He didn't even ask me what I eat or don't eat...he was just too eager to hand out the prescription.

*THANKS,*
*Max Greenfield*

Praise for The Blood Pressure Miracle

"Frank Mangano's new book The Blood Pressure Miracle is nothing short of a miracle. I regularly recommend it to all of my patients to help them lower their blood pressure and gain control of their lives. This invaluable tool is priceless in today's world of improper diet and stress."

*Steve G. Jones, M.Ed.*
*Clinical Hypnotherapist*
*www.gethypnosis.com*

"If you've already been diagnosed with high blood pressure, then it's urgent to take steps to lower it immediately. The Blood Pressure Miracle explains in simple terms the do's and don'ts of managing your blood pressure without outrageously-priced pharmacy drugs or suffering through dangerous side effects of harmful drugs. It is a must-read book that can save your life."

*Kent Sayre, Author*
*Unstoppable Confidence*
*www.unstoppable-confidence.com*

"High blood pressure, stroke and heart attack (the big three) often create a dependence on prescription drugs that have many side effects - often impotency and depression.

The fact is that you don't ever have to say the words, "Before my stroke (or heart attack)." Instead you can substitute the words, "Before I knew how to prevent and reverse the big three" with the application of the knowledge in Frank Mangano's book, "The Blood Pressure Miracle." That's because he lists and explains the most effective nutritional supplements and their dosages that can prevent and reverse high blood pressure.

While being in the nutritional field for over 20 years, I've seen the emergence of a true desire for what people can do to improve their health. We're taking care of our health now more than ever, and with available and easily accessible information such as this, we give ourselves the chance to recover gracefully and in a wholesome, healthy
fashion. This book is for men and women alike."

*Dr. Donna Schwontkowski*
*Chiropractic Physician,*
*Nutritionist/Master Herbalist*

# Contents

Foreword by Steve G. Jones, M.Ed. . . . . . . . . . . . . . . . . . . . . . . xiii
Acknowledgments. . . . . . . . . . . . . . . . . . . . . . . . . . . . . . . . . . . . xv
Introduction. . . . . . . . . . . . . . . . . . . . . . . . . . . . . . . . . . . . . . . xvii

**Chapter 1—What Is 'The Silent Killer'?** . . . . . . . . . . . . . . . . . . . . . 1
You Can't Control What You Can't Measure: How to Quickly and
  Easily Measure Your Blood Pressure . . . . . . . . . . . . . . . . . . . . . 2
Taking Your Own Blood Pressure . . . . . . . . . . . . . . . . . . . . . . . . 3
How to Read (and Understand) Your Blood Pressure Better Than
  Your Doctor . . . . . . . . . . . . . . . . . . . . . . . . . . . . . . . . . . . . . . 5
Pre-Hypertension vs. Hypertension: The No-Nonsense Scoop on
  What Is What . . . . . . . . . . . . . . . . . . . . . . . . . . . . . . . . . . . . . 6
Study: Lowering Weight Starts with Lowering Blood Pressure. . . . . . . . 7
Is High Blood Pressure Associated with Joint Pain? . . . . . . . . . . . . . 8
Your Ticket to an Early Grave: The Risks of NOT Slashing
  Your Blood Pressure . . . . . . . . . . . . . . . . . . . . . . . . . . . . . . . . 9
Heart Disease as a Result of Long-Term High Blood Pressure . . . . . . . 10
How Did You "Get" High Blood Pressure? . . . . . . . . . . . . . . . . . . . 11
How Are You Living? The Crucial Lifestyle Risk Factors . . . . . . . . . . 12
Is It Your Parent's Fault? Genetic Risk Factors . . . . . . . . . . . . . . . 14
Are Specific Genes Linked to High Blood Pressure? . . . . . . . . . . . . . 14
Chapter Summary. . . . . . . . . . . . . . . . . . . . . . . . . . . . . . . . . . . . 15

**Chapter 2—The Common Blood Pressure Solution: Prescription
  Medications and Why You Need to Avoid Them if Possible** . . . . . . . 17
What Your Doctor Wants to Prescribe to You and Why . . . . . . . . . . . . 18
The Dark Side of Prescription Drugs: The Side Effects That Could
  Make You Miserable . . . . . . . . . . . . . . . . . . . . . . . . . . . . . . . .

Kicking the Drug Habit: How to Free Yourself from High Prices and
    Miserable Side Effects . . . . . . . . . . . . . . . . . . . . . . . . . 22
Getting Your Doctor on Your Team . . . . . . . . . . . . . . . . . . . . 22
Chapter Summary . . . . . . . . . . . . . . . . . . . . . . . . . . . . . 23


**Chapter 3—My Handpicked Essential Vitamins, Minerals,
    and Herbs That Pass the "Mangano Quality Test"** . . . . . . . . . 25
The Power of Potassium . . . . . . . . . . . . . . . . . . . . . . . . . . 26
A Lesson About Lecithin . . . . . . . . . . . . . . . . . . . . . . . . . . 28
Calcium . . . . . . . . . . . . . . . . . . . . . . . . . . . . . . . . . . 28
Magnificent Magnesium . . . . . . . . . . . . . . . . . . . . . . . . . . 30
Keen for Quinoa . . . . . . . . . . . . . . . . . . . . . . . . . . . . . . 31
How Nature Made It: Natural Vitamin E vs. Synthetic . . . . . . . . . . 34
The Skinny on Omega-3 Fatty Acids (Fish Oils) . . . . . . . . . . . . . 35
Coenzyme Q10: What One-Third of Hypertension Patients Lack . . . . . 35
Supercharge Your Efforts with Coenzyme A . . . . . . . . . . . . . . . 36
Cleaning Up with Beta Glucan . . . . . . . . . . . . . . . . . . . . . . . 37
Making Sense of Selenium . . . . . . . . . . . . . . . . . . . . . . . . . 37
Bone Up on Bioflavonoids . . . . . . . . . . . . . . . . . . . . . . . . . 38
Fighting Heart Disease with Folic Acid and Vitamin B6 . . . . . . . . . 39
The L-Arginine Link . . . . . . . . . . . . . . . . . . . . . . . . . . . . 40
Heart-Healthy Herbs . . . . . . . . . . . . . . . . . . . . . . . . . . . . 41
The Strengthening Powers of Grape Seed Extract . . . . . . . . . . . . 42
The Right Food and Supplement Mix . . . . . . . . . . . . . . . . . . . 43
Daily Dosages of Beetroot Juice to Beat High Blood Pressure . . . . . . 44
Dark Chocolate and Your Lower Blood Pressure . . . . . . . . . . . . . 44
Boost Your Olive Oil Intake for Results . . . . . . . . . . . . . . . . . . 45
Your Choice of Herbal Supplements . . . . . . . . . . . . . . . . . . . . 46
Natural Alternatives: Homeopathy . . . . . . . . . . . . . . . . . . . . . 47
Chapter Summary . . . . . . . . . . . . . . . . . . . . . . . . . . . . . 48


**Chapter 4—Making Your Heart Love You** . . . . . . . . . . . . . . . 51
Trim the Flab, Stay in Shape, and Feel Great . . . . . . . . . . . . . . . 52
Taking the Mystery Out of Eating Right . . . . . . . . . . . . . . . . . . 53
Tips to Help with Fat Loss, High Blood Pressure, and Joint Pain . . . . . 55
The Mangano View on Meat . . . . . . . . . . . . . . . . . . . . . . . . 57
Where Sodium Belongs in Your Diet: The Answer Will Surprise You . . . 59
Knocking Hidden Sodium Out of Your Diet . . . . . . . . . . . . . . . . 61
Washing Away the Excess: The Role of Water . . . . . . . . . . . . . . . 62

Why Organic?. . . . . . . . . . . . . . . . . . . . . . . . . . . . . . . . . . . . . . . . . . 64
Top Ways We Sabotage Our Blood-Pressure-Lowering Efforts . . . . . . . . . 65
Chapter Summary . . . . . . . . . . . . . . . . . . . . . . . . . . . . . . . . . . . . . . . 67

**Chapter 5—Where the Rubber Meets the Road: Taking Action to**
    **Control and Manage Your Blood Pressure** . . . . . . . . . . . . . . . . . . . . . **69**
The Benefits of Exercise. . . . . . . . . . . . . . . . . . . . . . . . . . . . . . . . . . . 69
Start Dreaming About Lower Blood Pressure . . . . . . . . . . . . . . . . . . . 71
Reduce Your Stress to Reduce Your Blood Pressure. . . . . . . . . . . . . . . 72
Smell Your Way to Lower Blood Pressure. . . . . . . . . . . . . . . . . . . . . . 73
Eat Your Way to Lower Blood Pressure. . . . . . . . . . . . . . . . . . . . . . . . 74
Drink Your Way to Lower Blood Pressure. . . . . . . . . . . . . . . . . . . . . . 75
Listen Your Way to Lower Blood Pressure . . . . . . . . . . . . . . . . . . . . . 76
Reaping the Benefits of Meditation . . . . . . . . . . . . . . . . . . . . . . . . . . 77
Relax for Lower Blood Pressure: My Favorite Techniques . . . . . . . . . . . 78
The Truth About Yoga and Blood Pressure . . . . . . . . . . . . . . . . . . . . . 79
The Surefire Instant Calming Sequence . . . . . . . . . . . . . . . . . . . . . . . 79
Biofeedback for Lower Blood Pressure . . . . . . . . . . . . . . . . . . . . . . . . 80
Happiness Is Lower Blood Pressure. . . . . . . . . . . . . . . . . . . . . . . . . . . 81
Mapping Out Your Own Exercise Plan . . . . . . . . . . . . . . . . . . . . . . . . 82
Fitting Exercise into Your Everyday Life. . . . . . . . . . . . . . . . . . . . . . . 83
Chapter Summary . . . . . . . . . . . . . . . . . . . . . . . . . . . . . . . . . . . . . . . 84

**Chapter 6—The Sixty-Day Plan** . . . . . . . . . . . . . . . . . . . . . . . . . . . . . **85**
Adding Supplements. . . . . . . . . . . . . . . . . . . . . . . . . . . . . . . . . . . . . . 86
Menu Planning . . . . . . . . . . . . . . . . . . . . . . . . . . . . . . . . . . . . . . . . . 88
Exercise Plan. . . . . . . . . . . . . . . . . . . . . . . . . . . . . . . . . . . . . . . . . . . 88
Keeping Track. . . . . . . . . . . . . . . . . . . . . . . . . . . . . . . . . . . . . . . . . . 93
A Lifelong Change . . . . . . . . . . . . . . . . . . . . . . . . . . . . . . . . . . . . . . . 94

**References** . . . . . . . . . . . . . . . . . . . . . . . . . . . . . . . . . . . . . . . . . . . . . **97**
Books . . . . . . . . . . . . . . . . . . . . . . . . . . . . . . . . . . . . . . . . . . . . . . . . 97
Online Resources . . . . . . . . . . . . . . . . . . . . . . . . . . . . . . . . . . . . . . . 98

*About Frank Mangano*. . . . . . . . . . . . . . . . . . . . . . . . . . . . . . . . . . . *99*

# Foreword by Steve G. Jones, M.Ed.

It is truly an honor and a privilege to be writing a foreword for Frank Mangano's book The Blood Pressure Miracle. I first met Frank in 2003 when he approached me about my hypnotherapy products. I knew right away that both Frank and I could learn a lot from each other. And looking back, we truly have grown as business partners and friends both contributing to each other's success.

Frank is a leader and an advocate for natural health. He has changed thousands of lives through his products and I know for a fact that we will change thousands of lives through this powerful book on blood pressure. I know that he will change the lives of his readers because he helped me change my life.

I am constantly seeking Frank's advice concerning how to lead a healthier lifestyle. He has taught me how to make little changes in my life and I have learned that little changes can produce major results. From Frank, I have learned which foods will enhance my overall health and I have noticed major changes in my energy level, my ability to focus, and my fitness.

Frank Mangano is my mentor in natural health. I seek his advice on which products to buy that will help me lead a more natural, healthy, and chemical free lifestyle. I am truly astounded by his wealth of knowledge.

When I started reading this book, I realized I could not put it down. I had no idea that blood pressure could affect the body in so many different ways. In my opinion, Frank has a knack for simplifying complex medical concepts and delivering a total, no-nonsense solution that will greatly benefit you. I've reviewed this book and I give it my highest recommendation.

Reading this book, one can tell that Frank has done his research. He has dedicated his life to spreading the word about blood pressure. I believe so strongly in The Blood Pressure Miracle that I recommend this book to all of my clients who are suffering from high blood pressure, joint pain, and even those who are having difficulties losing weight. This book shows concrete evidence that there is a high correlation between high blood pressure and inability to lose weight.

I have never been diagnosed with high blood pressure, but after reading this book I realize that I must take an active role in keeping my blood pressure in the normal range. I want to protect my heart so that I can live a longer and healthier life. After reading this book I am sure you as the reader will also feel motivated to make changes in your life. It gives me great pleasure to know that you're interested in controlling your blood pressure and you do not have to rely on prescription drugs to control it for you. The fact that you're reading these words now indicates that you have decided to take charge of your health.

Steve G. Jones M.Ed.
Clinical Hypnotherapist
http://www.gethypnosis.com

# Acknowledgments

First and foremost, I am thankful for the support of my mom, Patricia, my dad, Frank and my brother, Danny. They provided continuous encouragement throughout this book project. They believed in me and in this book. I love them dearly. I want to give a very special thanks to Kim Wierman and Ben Carder for assisting me in my research for this book. Special thanks to Strategic Book Publishing for taking on this project. Thanks also to Ron Reale, who provided editorial assistance to this book. I want to thank Paul Mascetta, Michael Maloney and Steve G. Jones for their support during this book project. Last, but certainly not least, I am grateful to God for giving me this opportunity to help others.

# Introduction

Congratulations! You are truly a genius for purchasing *The Blood Pressure Miracle!*

Here's why: Most people WANT to slash their high blood pressure but they never do anything about it. You are different, and for that, I commend you. You took action to invest in your health because you understand how important it is to get your high blood pressure under control. It is very likely that you can achieve your goal by following the "Mangano" method, while remaining under the care of your physician.

*The Blood Pressure Miracle* has a simple, easy-to-follow solution for lowering blood pressure without costly drug prescriptions, or suffering through the miserable side effects of blood-pressure-controlling drugs. Realize this: You don't need every solution under the sun to lower your blood pressure. *The Blood Pressure Miracle* doesn't contain 367 new-fangled ways to drop blood pressure. This book merely contains one good one. And my friend, that's all you need. This is the last resource on lowering your high blood pressure that you're ever going to need.

The majority of my customers are wonderful and they love *The Blood Pressure Miracle*. I've had a handful of self-proclaimed know-it-alls who have read *The Blood Pressure Miracle* and said they already knew everything in it... yet they still had high blood pressure! Here's my point: If you study this book and apply what you learn, you'll get results. I don't know how to say it any plainer or simpler than that. If you do nothing, you'll get zero results. Apply what you learn.

If you're one of those people who studies endlessly about high blood pressure, but doesn't do a darn thing, then you're going to hate this program. It's not a magic pill that will do all the work for you, nor is it meant to sit in your library just for the fun of it. It is meant to give you applicable solutions to your high blood pressure.

Think about this: Would you rather be a know-it-all about high blood pressure and still have high blood pressure or would you rather know all you need to know (which you'll get in this program) and have lower, healthy blood pressure? I would personally choose to know enough and get results than know everything but still suffer from a potentially deadly problem.

Now hear me out. What I'm about to say is very grim, yet I need to remind you of the grave importance of treating your high blood pressure. Here it is: Some of you with high blood pressure who are reading this right now may face serious health risks as a direct consequence of your high blood pressure... if you don't get it treated. Prevent those health risks by lowering your blood pressure now.

While this book presents a potential treatment for lowering your blood pressure, you should be under the care of your doctor as you study it inside and out, and then apply it.

## GETTING YOUR BEARINGS: A RAPID, EASY INTRODUCTION TO HIGH BLOOD PRESSURE

The fact that you purchased this book to lower your blood pressure levels tells me that you or someone you know has been told they have high blood pressure. The reason I know you have been "told" this is that no one really knows when their blood pressure is high or approaching dangerously high readings. There are no symptoms and you feel just fine. You are basically in good health otherwise. So how can it be that your blood pressure is high?

High blood pressure, officially known as hypertension, has inherited the nickname of "Silent Killer", and for good reason. According to the American Heart Association, 20 percent of adult Americans have high blood pressure. Of that number, 30 percent don't even know it. How could someone not know they have such a potentially serious condition? Unless their blood pressure read high during regular medical check-ups, there was most likely no indication that they were suffering from this medical condition.

There are many prescription drugs that can be taken for treating high blood pressure. Unfortunately, it is not a condition that can be cured or even prevented. This is mostly because medical professionals don't know exactly what causes it. However, they do know that there are factors such as heredity, body type, lifestyle, diet, and exercise that contribute to the onset of hypertension. The good news is that high blood pressure can be managed and lowered by improving the flow of blood through the arteries. Even better news is that this does not have to necessarily be achieved by taking prescription drugs. There are foods, supplements, exercises, and stress-reducing practices that can work together to lower blood pressure in most adults.

Why bother with all this if you feel just fine? The answer may take years of untreated high blood pressure before you really have the proof of the damage hypertension can cause. While high blood pressure doesn't make you feel bad right now, it can cause serious conditions such as strokes, heart attacks, and other types of heart disease if left untreated. The extra work the heart must do to push blood through the body will eventually take its toll on the heart and arteries. This can adversely affect not only your well-being, but also the length of your life.

*The Blood Pressure Miracle* is intended to teach you a few important facts about hypertension and the ways in which you can manage it naturally; that is to say without the use of prescription drugs and their undesirable side effects. It will explain why natural is a better alternative to prescription drugs. You will also learn that while you can't always predict or prevent hypertension, you can surely postpone its onset and control it through diet, exercise, and a regime of supplement usage that provides heart-healthy benefits.

You have taken the first step to ensuring you have a healthy heart well into your old age. By taking the preventative measures now and keeping your blood pressure under control, you are setting yourself up for lifelong habits that will keep your heart healthy and let you enjoy good heart health now and years down the road. You can have all this without a lifelong dependency on prescription medications. Read on to take that proactive and natural approach to lowering your blood pressure and protecting your heart.

# 1

# What Is 'The Silent Killer'?

In the simplest terms, blood pressure is the amount of force the blood puts on the arteries as it passes through. This force can be greater in some people than others. When the walls of your arteries have a greater force on them than is considered safe and healthy, you are said to have high blood pressure.

Why is too much force unhealthy? When someone has excessive force put on their arteries, they don't feel it or even notice any symptoms. That is why maybe comparing it to something you can physically feel will help you understand its impact.

An analogy of a balloon can be used to illustrate what happens to your heart when there is too much force of blood through the arteries. Pretend you are blowing up the type of balloon clowns use to make animals with during children's birthday parties. Those balloons are long and skinny and can be compared to your arteries. If you have ever tried blowing air into one of those balloons, you know it takes a lot of force. Your cheeks puff out, you get red in the face, and you may even get a little light-headed as you try to force air into the balloon. You basically have to work so hard at getting the air through, that your lungs have to work overtime, causing those uncomfortable symptoms.

The same is true with blood pressure. When it takes so much force to push blood through the arteries, your heart has to work overtime. It doesn't get to rest, either. When you stop blowing the balloon, your lungs go back to a normal workload very quickly. In the case of high blood pressure, the heart never gets a rest or gets to return to a lighter workload.

The impact of this effort is an overworked, underappreciated heart! This makes that vital organ enlarged from flexing its pumping muscles so hard for so long. An enlarged heart, over-forced arteries, and diminished blood flow are what lead to other illness, disease, and degeneration of organs. This is why it is so important to keep blood pressure under control.

## YOU CAN'T CONTROL WHAT YOU CAN'T MEASURE: HOW TO QUICKLY AND EASILY MEASURE YOUR BLOOD PRESSURE

From the time you were a child every doctor's visit included having your blood pressure taken. This may not be something you ever really paid attention to since there were probably no adverse readings. The blood pressure cuff that was wrapped around your arm and the little bulb that was used to pump the cuff until it got tighter and tighter may have fascinated you.

The same equipment is used in most doctors' offices today, as it was twenty and thirty years ago. There are many hospitals that have automated versions of the Velcro-closed cuff that stays wrapped around your upper arm and periodically tightens to take a reading. Other than that, the blood-pressure-reading equipment hasn't changed much. However, what healthcare professionals are doing with the results has.

When a blood pressure reading is taken, the nurse uses the cuff to constrict the arm so that he or she can hear two specific times that the heart beats. The first reading is a measurement of how much pressure is put on the artery as the heart makes a beat. As the nurse tightens the cuff and listens with a stethoscope, there comes a point when the heartbeat can be heard. That is the systolic pressure.

Next, as the nurse releases the pressure, there comes a time when the heartbeat can no longer be heard. This is referred to as the diastolic pressure, and is the force on the arteries in between heartbeats when the heart is relaxed. That is why the final reading is one number written on top of another. This is then verbalized as "110 over 75" or written 110/75 on your chart. The gauge is actually measuring millimeters of mercury.

## *Terms:*

***Systolic pressure:*** The amount of force on the arteries as the heart beats and pushes the blood through, the top number in your blood pressure reading.

***Diastolic pressure:*** The amount of force of blood on the arteries as the heart relaxes between beats, the bottom number in your blood pressure reading.

## TAKING YOUR OWN BLOOD PRESSURE

Knowledge is power, and the best way to maintain a good quality of life is the knowledge of what your blood pressure is *before* the good doctor knows. Knowing this may spare you from having to take unnecessary—and unwanted—medications.

According to research done on the topic, a number of people get high blood pressure readings due to a phenomenon called "white coat" hypertension. This is where a man or woman fears what his or her own blood pressure reading will be, causing stress levels to rise. This in turn causes inaccurate readings and possibly inaccurate hypertension diagnoses.

The research conducted on this reaction involved 430 patients with hypertension, each randomly assigned to either office-measurement or self-measurement. Researchers found that at each visit the self-measurement group consistently had lower blood pressure readings than the office-measurement group. This made them more likely to be able to reduce or stop their blood pressure medication treatments, and their blood pressure treatments were less costly ($4,147 versus $3,023 per 100 patients per month).

Though self-measurement shouldn't replace office-reading measurements, self-measurement allows one to pinpoint signs of pre-hypertension. It can also help to minimize excessive, unnecessary medical costs due to improper diagnoses that result from false measurements.

Ideally, you can have someone else at home take your blood pressure. However, if you're all by your lonesome, be aware that taking your blood pressure can't be done in a loud room or while you're distracted. It requires careful attention and a piqued ear.

1. First, feel for your pulse on the inside part of your arm, the opposite side of where your elbow bends.

2. With your arm straightened, palm up, and the sphygmomanometer (i.e. the technical term for what's used to measure your blood pressure) reader facing you, attach the blood pressure cuff right above the bend in the elbow, around the bicep.

3. Next, place the stethoscope's disc right where you felt for your pulse earlier—around the middle part of your arm where it bends. Make sure it is snug against your arm and that the bottom of the disc is not touching the cuff part. Put the earpieces of the stethoscope in your ears.

4. Squeeze the pump until the cuff is good and tight around your arm; it's usually tight enough when the arrow on the sphygmomanometer is 30 mmHg beyond the point where you can no longer feel or hear your pulse—between 180 and 200 mmHg.

5. Once it's tight enough, *slowly* release the air in the cuff with the release valve.

6. Here is where you really need to look and listen. While you're slowly releasing the air, listen for the first beat you hear in the stethoscope's earpieces, that is your systolic pressure; you'll know what number it is by watching the gauge to see what number the scale is showing at the first sound.

7. Now you need to listen for the last sound you hear. The last beat you hear in the stethoscope is the sound of blood flowing through your veins. The less constricted the blood vessels are, the harder it is to hear. Remembering to watch the gauge and still slowly releasing the valve, listen carefully because it will be faint. This is your diastolic pressure reading.

This will take some practice; so don't get frustrated if you're having trouble after the first several tries. Practice makes perfect.

Once you've mastered it, keep the following things in mind:

• Try to take your blood pressure around the same time every day; what you're doing at any given time can affect the accuracy of the reading.

• If you've just exercised, take your blood pressure at least a half hour after your cool down.

• Try to relax. Stress, anger, or frustration can cause inaccurate readings.

## HOW TO READ (AND UNDERSTAND) YOUR BLOOD PRESSURE BETTER THAN YOUR DOCTOR

So you leave the doctor's office with these numbers in your head. What exactly do they mean? Guidelines from the National Heart, Lung & Blood Institute of the National Institute of Health reveal that the ideal blood pressure reading is when the systolic, or top number, in the reading is less than 120 millimeters of mercury (mmHg) and the diastolic, or bottom number, reads less than 80 mmHg.

For adults, there is a range of blood pressure levels that are considered normal and healthy. The following chart illustrates those ranges.

**Blood Pressure Levels Measured in Millimeters of Mercury (mmHg)**

| Classification | Systolic (top number) | | Diastolic (bottom number) |
|---|---|---|---|
| Normal | Less than 120 | And | Less than 80 |
| Pre-hypertension (early warning stage) | 120–139 | Or | 80–89 |
| Stage 1 Hypertension (high blood pressure) | 140–159 | Or | 90–99 |
| Stage 2 Hypertension (severely high blood pressure) | Greater than or equal to 160 | Or | Greater than or equal to 100 |

Source: Guide of Lowering Blood Pressure from the National Heart, Lung, and Blood Institute (NHLBI)

When one number is high and the other is "normal," the high number is used to categorize the entire blood pressure reading. It is an "and/or" type of situation. For example, a measurement of 135/80 has both numbers as indicators of hypertension. However, the stage is considered stage 1 since the higher of the two numbers is in that category. A reading of 120/95 is still stage 1, even though the systolic reading (120) is within the pre-hypertension range.

## PRE-HYPERTENSION VS. HYPERTENSION: THE NO-NONSENSE SCOOP ON WHAT IS WHAT

Pre-hypertension is classified as a blood pressure reading of between 120 and 139 for the systolic measurement and between 80 and 89 for the diastolic reading. If you are getting your blood pressure checked regularly and your readings are consistently within this range, now is the time to take serious action to keep it under control.

Many people at a pre-hypertension stage are given a kind of forewarning that may mean the difference between the lifelong use of medication or not. Since this book is intended to teach you how to manage your blood pressure without medication, starting at the pre-hypertension stage, it gives you an even better advantage. By following the recommendations of this book and your doctor, chances are promising that you will never get to the point of stage 1 or stage 2 hypertension.

At the very least, you can postpone the onset, reducing the length of time your heart has to work hard at pumping blood through the arteries. For every year that you can keep the pre-hypertension readings from climbing, you prolong the time your heart is working at an optimal workload. The chain reaction carries through. By controlling the pre-hypertension, you control the impact on the heart, which in turn keeps the heart healthy and postpones or prevents other more serious conditions. We'll go into what the consequences of not lowering your blood pressure can mean in the next section.

Hypertension, on the other hand, means your blood pressure levels have already reached the higher numbered readings of this condition. While you can't cure yourself of hypertension, you can control it. By reducing your blood pressure even from stage 1 hypertension to pre-hypertension, or from stage 2 down to stage 1, you are improving your health.

The method to lowering the pressure in a way that does not involve the use of prescription medications is what this book is all about. Now we'll get into just why lowering your blood pressure is so important.

## STUDY: LOWERING WEIGHT STARTS WITH LOWERING BLOOD PRESSURE

Why is it so important? Let me count the ways. For starters, lowering your blood pressure can actually increase your ability to lose weight and help eliminate joint pain. Most people know that being overweight can lead to high blood pressure and joint pain, but now we know that the other way around is true, too.

In fact, you'll soon understand how lowering your blood pressure can cause you to lose weight easier and reduce, or even eliminate, your joint pain!

How?

I want you to pay very close attention to what you're about to learn. When you look at the overall picture of this study, it simply means that *high blood pressure can lead to greater cravings for carbohydrates, which means less fat burning.* According to the following study, biology dictates that a body with high blood pressure craves more carbohydrates.

There was an eye-opening study conducted by researchers at the Washington University School of Medicine in St. Louis. This study can be found in the *Journal of Nuclear Cardiology.*

This research shows that the heart muscle in diabetic people relies heavily on fat to use as energy. Fat *is* useful as fuel. However, burning the fat turns into an extraordinary requirement for oxygen in diabetics and the heart becomes more susceptible to the reduced oxygen levels associated with coronary artery blockage.

Researchers have also concluded that a heart not suffering from diabetes, but afflicted with muscle thickening due to hypertension has an energy metabolism in the opposite direction. These individuals *do not use fat for energy.*

Lisa de las Fuentes, M.D., who led the research, states that a heart with hypertrophy (muscle thickening) gets a lower amount of energy due to the reduced fat metabolism. This, in turn, *leads these individuals to rely on a larger carbohydrate intake.*

"Carbohydrates produce less energy per molecule than fatty acids," she says. "With hypertrophy, the heart has a higher energy demand because there's more muscle to feed. With less fat metabolism, a greater reliance on carbohydrates may represent a shift to a less-efficient fuel."

This was a human study on patients who had high blood pressure that resulted in muscle thickening of the left ventricle, which is the largest chamber of the heart, and is responsible for pumping blood throughout the body. The study concluded that the higher the muscle mass of the heart with hypertrophy, the less ability it has to burn fat.

**The study helps to show that high blood pressure can actually deter you from burning fat and thus prevent you from losing weight.**

## IS HIGH BLOOD PRESSURE ASSOCIATED WITH JOINT PAIN?

Another reason why lowering high blood pressure is so important is the relationship high blood pressure has with joint pain. This theory was tested and proven by a recent study done at Brigham and Women's Hospital, a Harvard University research and teaching facility. The study, published by the American Heart Associations's *Circulation* looked at the relationship between joint pain, specifically arthritis, and hypertension or high blood pressure. The results showed that there is a correlation between the two. People with arthritis have a lower life expectancy and often suffer from complications of heart disease and high blood pressure.

The study found that high blood pressure is often found among those who suffer with arthritis. The risk for heart attack becomes greater the longer the patient has the increased joint pain. This may partly be due to the fact that the inflammation associated with joint pain may be caused by an accumulation of white blood cells, which can, in turn, restrict the arteries. High blood pressure can make matters worse in these cases.

While those with normal blood pressure levels may not put any additional stress on the joints, those with elevated blood pressure just might. High blood pressure can put undue stress on most parts of the body, including organs such as the heart.

The study examined more than 114,000 women. However, according to Daniel Solomon, the assistant professor of medicine at Harvard Medical School, "There is no reason to believe that this relationship would not be seen in men as well."

Additionally, it is often the case that those with joint pain have restricted movements and reduced physical activity. This can hinder several things, including low cholesterol, weight control, and heart disease. It seems that these factors work together to create a situation that can cause additional health problems. The study notes similar testing done in Canada, which found that people with rheumatoid arthritis died an average of seventeen years sooner than the average life expectancy for the Canadian population.

Indeed, it seems likely that high blood pressure can affect many parts of the body, including the joints. Reducing high blood pressure can help to reduce associated risks, including heart attacks. It may be possible to reduce joint inflammation when less pressure is constantly put on them.

One should conclude from this study that when blood pressure is lowered, there is less joint pain. This may partially be due to the blood having a much easier time circulating through narrow passages such as in the joints. It can be noted, that lowering your blood pressure can help alleviate joint pain.

Of course, lowering the blood pressure has an important medical impact on many other parts of the body as well. Those who can lower their blood pressure have a significant reduction in the risk of heart attack and stroke.

## YOUR TICKET TO AN EARLY GRAVE: THE RISKS OF NOT SLASHING YOUR BLOOD PRESSURE

Reducing weight and lessening joint pain are just some of the important reasons to lower your blood pressure. However, the biggest and most important reason to lower high blood pressure is to reduce the negative effect that added force on the arteries has on other areas of the body. This includes various organs and systems. This effect may take years, even decades to manifest itself.

But a look at the long-term effects of untreated high blood pressure leads doctors to take a very proactive role in treating hypertension.

## Atherosclerosis

One very serious condition that can result from years of untreated high blood pressure is atherosclerosis. This is a condition that is usually related to high cholesterol, but is contributed to by untreated high blood pressure. Many of the lifestyle changes associated with lowering cholesterol also apply to lowering high blood pressure. Atherosclerosis, which is sometimes referred to as a hardening of the arteries, is when the arteries are clogged and blood flow becomes restricted. When the blood is pushed through the arteries with a greater force, as in a hypertension patient, this also adds to the damage of the artery lining. Damaged vessels are more likely to form deposits of fat and other types of buildup that lead to atherosclerosis.

Hardening of the arteries in the heart leads to heart failure and most likely death. A hardening of the blood vessels supplying the kidneys leads to kidney failure, as well as all other illness related to non-functioning kidneys.

### Aneurysm and Stroke

Another serious result of hypertension is a weakening of the arteries that can lead to an aneurysm. This type of rupture in the blood vessel causes the vessels that supply blood to the brain to have sudden bleeding outside the vessel. These are the precursors to the more serious, life-threatening conditions of stroke and heart attack.

## HEART DISEASE AS A RESULT OF LONG-TERM HIGH BLOOD PRESSURE

Heart disease results from high blood pressure in a roundabout way. High blood pressure creates a damaging buildup in the arteries and can cause them to become blocked or weakened. This can lead to a heart attack.

Another equally serious condition is heart failure. The formal name of heart failure, or stiffening of damaged arteries, is Hypertensive Heart Disease. When the walls in the left ventricle of the heart, which is the lower left chamber, become thick, they also stiffen. This makes it difficult for the heart to pump blood throughout the body. When the heart has to work so hard just to pump enough blood to the various parts of the body, it can lead to heart failure. The heart simply can't do what it needs to do.

## HOW DID YOU "GET" HIGH BLOOD PRESSURE?

Although the healthcare profession doesn't claim to know the real cause of high blood pressure, they do know that certain factors contribute to it. Since the risk factors are so easily identified, it's simple to determine which ones might apply to you. Then, you can try to head off the onset of high blood pressure by making changes in your life in the areas over which you have control. You can also manage your blood pressure by managing the risk factors.

These risk factors can be separated into three basic categories: lifestyle; heredity or genetics, including body type; and age. First, if you aren't concerned about having high blood pressure, maybe you should take a look at these statistics from the American Heart Association:

- High blood pressure was listed on death certificates as the primary cause of death of 54,707 Americans in 2004. High blood pressure was listed as a primary or contributing cause of death in about 300,000 of the more than 2.4 million U.S. deaths in 2004.

- About 73 million people in the United States age twenty and older have high blood pressure.

- One in three U.S. adults has high blood pressure.

- Twenty-eight percent of people with high blood pressure don't know they have it.

- Of all people with high blood pressure, 71.8 percent are aware of their condition, 61.4 percent are under treatment, 35.1 percent have it under control, and 64.9 percent do not.

- The cause of 90 to 95 percent of the cases of high blood pressure isn't known; however, high blood pressure is easily detected and usually controllable.

- From 1994 to 2004 the death rate from high blood pressure increased 26.6 percent, and the actual number of deaths rose 56.1 percent.

- People with less education and low income levels tend to have higher levels of blood pressure.

- The 2004 overall death rate from high blood pressure was 18.1. Death rates were 15.7 for white males, 14.5 for white females, 51.0 for black males, and 40.9 for black females.

## HOW ARE YOU LIVING? THE CRUCIAL LIFESTYLE RISK FACTORS

The biggest contributors to high blood pressure over which you have at least some control all relate to lifestyle choices.

### Obesity and Diet

Obesity and the excessive consumption of fatty foods is a key contributor to high blood pressure. Maintaining a normal weight for your age and height is important in preventing many different health issues. To keep blood pressure in check, your body mass index (BMI) should be in the range of 18.5 and 24.9.

Diet also contributes to controlling blood pressure, even if you are not overweight. Reducing sodium is key. Ideally, you should not have more than 2,400 mg of sodium per day. This is a very small amount—the equivalent of about one teaspoon! Many processed foods use sodium to preserve them, so even if you don't ever grab the saltshaker, your sodium intake could be high without you even realizing it.

### Lack of Exercise

Lack of exercise also affects blood pressure negatively, especially if you are in a high-risk group due to age or heredity. Exercise, especially cardiovascular workouts, increases the heart rate, which helps maintain good blood pressure levels. At least twenty to thirty minutes of exercise each day is ideal. A lack of exercise can also lead to obesity, one of the consequences we've already discussed.

## Smoking and Alcohol Consumption

The "little sins" of smoking and drinking can lead to big problems with blood pressure. Although some will claim that scientific evidence supports the idea that moderate amounts of alcohol have positive benefits, there really is no long-term proof. The biggest problem with alcohol consumption is that many people have different definitions of "moderate." The National Institute of Health has set a guideline for men of no more than three drinks per day. For women and smaller men, this number drops to two. While lower levels of alcohol consumption may not contribute to high blood pressure, this type of drinking does lead to other unhealthy conditions.

There is no question in anyone's mind that smoking is unhealthy. Even the tobacco producers know this. What you may not know is how smoking affects blood pressure. Again, it is the arteries that are under attack when you smoke. Each time you inhale, you are causing the arteries to constrict. In addition, the nicotine in tobacco acts to increase blood pressure as long as it is in the body. If you are a continuous smoker with an addiction to nicotine, then your nicotine levels are so high that your blood pressure is elevated to a dangerous amount. And let's face it, if heart disease from high blood pressure doesn't kill you, then lung cancer probably will. It is never healthy to smoke, even just a little!

## Stress

Mental stress and physical stress are two different things. When we exercise, we are putting a good type of stress on our circulatory system. This exercises the heart, lungs, and muscles in a way that strengthens the entire body and helps it resist disease and injury.

Mental stress from a hectic, out-of-control lifestyle is not healthy. Everyone experiences stress periodically but then returns back to a more comfortable, normal level. When those stress levels never get a break, that is when trouble begins.

Mental stress, as well as physical stress has the ability to raise blood pressure temporarily. When stress is ongoing, so is the higher blood pressure level. By never giving your stress level a chance to recover, you are keeping your blood pressure raised. Over time, this can cause the serious health issues related to uncontrolled blood pressure.

## IS IT YOUR PARENT'S FAULT? GENETIC RISK FACTORS

Family history and heredity play a very significant role in whether you will have high blood pressure at some point in your life. If you are of African descent, then that risk is even higher. It is not known why African-Americans have more problems with high blood pressure than others. It is only known that their blood pressure can reach severely high levels and at an earlier age than Caucasians.

If you have a parent, grandparent, brother, or sister with high blood pressure, it is a good idea to monitor yours regularly. Even if you have a healthy lifestyle consisting of good eating habits and exercise and you don't smoke or drink excessively, you still may be at risk if there are others in your family with hypertension.

Body type also plays a role in your likelihood of having high blood pressure. Genetics are the reason we are either pear-shaped (with larger hips and smaller waists) like many women, or apple-shaped (with a bigger gut) like some men. The reason more men are likely to have high blood pressure than women is that men tend to gain weight in their middle where women gain in the hips. This generalization doesn't exempt one gender over the other. It is just known that when extra weight is carried in the middle, it leads to more heart problems than those who are bottom heavy.

Finally, age is a major contributor to high blood pressure. It is not, however, considered a healthy, normal part of aging. It just means that many older people have elevated blood pressure readings. This may be due to older people not having a diet with the nutrients that support good blood pressure or because as we age we may become more sedentary. Both diet and exercise play a major role in maintaining good blood pressure. There is no reason to stop these healthy habits as we age, and in fact, they become even more important in maintaining a good quality of life.

## ARE SPECIFIC GENES LINKED TO HIGH BLOOD PRESSURE?

While findings are far from conclusive, a recent study suggests having a specific type of gene may explain why some people are predisposed to hypertension. It's called STK39, or the serine/threonine kinase gene. When researchers from the University of Maryland analyzed DNA samples from about 600 people and analyzed how that gene compared to approximately 100,000 other genetic variants linked to blood pressure levels, they found that people with this particular gene variant had blood pressure levels higher than those who didn't have the STK39 gene in their DNA. To confirm their results, they performed similar tests on four other groups of participants (all Caucasian) around the country. Those results confirmed their original set of findings—that people with the STK39 gene had slightly higher blood pressure levels than those without the gene variant.

The STK39 gene plays a role in how the kidneys utilize salt in the digestive process. And as we all know, salt is a key contributor to hypertension. The researchers believe that approximately 20 percent of the American public has this type of gene.

## CHAPTER SUMMARY

Since you now know that there are many factors that contribute to high blood pressure, you also know that there are proactive approaches to keeping blood pressure readings at a healthy level.

Diet and exercise can and will keep blood pressure in check and usually just as well as prescription medications. It takes a commitment to controlling what you can control. The odds are in your favor, even if you have genetic factors that put you at a higher risk.

The next chapter describes the most commonly used treatment for high blood pressure—prescription drugs. It is important to understand how and why these are prescribed in your effort to have a drug-free approach to managing your blood pressure.

# 2

# The Common Blood Pressure Solution: Prescription Medications and Why You Need to Avoid Them if Possible

High blood pressure medications are a booming business among drug manufacturers. With millions of Americans in need of treatment to help lower their blood pressure, there is no shortage of prescriptions available to help them.

There are problems with high blood pressure medications that go beyond side effects and cost. Some prescriptions are actually very inexpensive and do a reasonable job of controlling moderate cases of stage 1 hypertension. The number one reason to try to manage your blood pressure naturally lies in lifestyle. Once prescribed a medication for high blood pressure, it is extremely unlikely that you will ever again be able to live without it. Not impossible, just unlikely and difficult.

Because of the nature of high blood pressure medications, it can take years before the right combination and dosage actually begin working to effectively lower blood pressure. The medications usually work in combination, meaning you will probably be treated with two or even three different prescriptions.

If you are already on blood pressure-lowering medication, it is important that you do not make any adjustments to your prescribed treatment without continuous monitoring and care by your doctor. The inherent design of the drugs prescribed causes reactions in the body that can be harmful if stopped abruptly. Understanding how these drugs work in the body and how they are intended to lower blood pressure will help you understand the kind of care you should take in making a change to a drug-free treatment.

## WHAT YOUR DOCTOR WANTS TO PRESCRIBE TO YOU AND WHY

The goal of prescription drugs in the treatment of hypertension is to lower blood pressure. When the blood pressure is lowered, the heart works at a more desirable level and remains healthier.

All the prescription drugs used for lowering blood pressure can be broken down into general categories by how they work:

- By removing extra fluid and undesirable salt from the body

- By slowing down the heartbeat

- By relaxing and/or widening blood vessels

There are categories of drugs that accomplish each of these effects. For example, diuretics (water pills) work with the kidneys to flush out excess fluid and fluid-retaining salt so that there is a better flow of blood through the vessels. Blood volume is actually lowered, which in turn lowers blood pressure. This type of medication is most often used when systolic (top) readings are high.

One commonly prescribed medication for this is called hydrochlorothiazide. It has many brand names such as Carozine, Diaqua, Esidrix, and HydroDiuril. This medication is often prescribed with others in the treatment of high blood pressure.

One of the worst side effects of taking a diuretic to manage blood pressure is that by flushing the body of the sodium and excessive fluid, you are also flushing the body of some minerals and nutrients that specifically help maintain good blood pressure levels. Other side effects can include dizziness, muscle cramps, and weakness (probably from the loss of potassium), all the way to the more serious side effects of abnormal bleeding, bruising, and irregular heartbeats.

## THE DARK SIDE OF PRESCRIPTION DRUGS: THE SIDE EFFECTS THAT COULD MAKE YOU MISERABLE

The chart on the following page summarizes the categories of blood pressure medications most commonly used today. The chart will show their classification, intended effect on the body, and some of the more common names.

As you will see by this chart, there are some pretty undesirable side effects that can come from the use of these medications. Sometimes you end up needing a medication to treat the side effect of the first medication. Before you know it, you are a walking medicine cabinet.

Symptoms are the body's way of telling us that something is not right. When we cover up the symptom with one medication after another, it is like putting a Band-Aid on a cut that needs stitches and hoping it won't scar. What you really need to do is treat the condition that is causing the symptom.

This is where the treatment of high blood pressure is tricky. Since there usually are no symptoms until another part of the body has been affected, lowering high blood pressure can be neglected until there is a major problem that could require surgery on the heart or arteries, or even result in death.

To avoid simply covering up high blood pressure as a bandage would a wound, you need to treat it from within, at the core of the nutritional and health issues that have caused it. Here is how the sixty-day plan comes into play. It works to improve health in such a core way that the root causes (other than heredity) are significantly reduced, thereby reducing blood pressure.

Another huge problem with prescription medications in the treatment of high blood pressure is that it is difficult to tell what blood vessel issues you

| Category Name | What It Does | Common Medications | Negative Side Effects |
|---|---|---|---|
| **Diuretics** Thiazide, Loop, Potassium-sparing, Other | Also known as water pills, these remove excess salt and water from the body and reduce blood volume | Thiazide generic and corresponding brands: chlorthalidone (Clorpres, Tenoretic, Thalitone), chlorothiazide (Diuril), hydrochlorothiazide (Capozide, Dyazide, Hyzaar, Lopressor HCT, Maxzide), indapamide (Lozol) <br> Loop generic and corresponding brands: bumetanide (Bumex), furosemide (Lasix), torsemide (Demadex) <br> Potassium-sparing generic and corresponding brands: amiloride, spironolactone (Aldactone), triamterene (Dyazide, Maxzide) <br> Other generic and corresponding brands: metolazone (Diulo, Zaroxolyn) | Increased thirst; increased urination for a few days after beginning medicine; reduced levels of potassium (heightened levels of potassium in potassium-sparing diuretics, which may lead to cardiac arrest due to abnormal heart rhythms); magnesium and sodium in blood; increased levels of uric acid, calcium, blood sugar (which may complicate control of diabetes), and cholesterol; weakness; impotence; dehydration; dry mouth; tooth decay; interaction with other medicines, like NSAIDs, cholesterol-lowering drugs, and lithium, a medicine used to treat certain mental illnesses; cramps; muscle paralysis |
| **Vasodilators** | Directly relaxes muscles in the blood vessel walls to open vessels | Generic and corresponding brands: clonidine (Catapres), guanabenz, guanadrel, guanfacine (Tenex), hydralazine, methyldopa (Aldomet), minoxidil | Fainting; rapid heartbeat; irregular heartbeat; headache; fluid retention; gastrointestinal disturbances (hydralazine only); hair growth (minoxidil only); very low blood pressure; drowsiness; dry mouth; impotence; fatigue; rapid return of high blood pressure if medicines are stopped suddenly; skin irritation |
| **Alpha blockers** | Relaxes tight blood vessels by reducing nerve impulses to allow for easier blood flow | Generic and corresponding brands: doxazosin (Cardura), prazosin (Minipress), terazosin (Hytrin), tamsulosin (Flomax), alfuzosin (Uroxatral) | Pronounced low blood pressure; dizziness (especially when rising from a sitting position); headache; pounding heartbeat; nausea; weakness; weight gain; may increase the risk of heart failure with long-term use |
| **Beta blockers** | Decreases heart rate and the amount of blood pushed though vessels with each beat. Also relaxes the blood vessels for easier blood flow | Generic and corresponding brands: acebutolol (Sectral), carvedilol (Coreg,) atenolol (Tenormin), betaxolol (Kerlone), labetalol (Normodyne, Trandate), metoprolol (Lopressor, Toprol XL), nadolol (Corgard), penbutolol (Levatol), pindolol (Visken), propranolol (Inderal), timolol | Lowered HDL (good) cholesterol; increased blood sugar levels; impotence; rapid heart rate if stopped suddenly; nightmares; limited endurance of a person who exercises (because they slow the heart rate); some beta blockers increase asthma symptoms |

| Category Name | What It Does | Common Medications | Negative Side Effects |
|---|---|---|---|
| **Alpha-beta blockers** | Combination of alpha and beta blockers—reduces nerve impulses and slows heart beat | Same as alpha blockers and beta blockers | Similar symptoms of both alpha and beta blockers |
| **ARBs** | (Formally known as Angiotensin II Receptor Blockers). Relaxes and widens blood vessels, thereby making it easier for the heart to pump blood by keeping out Angiotensin II. Increases release of sodium and water into urine | Generic and corresponding brands: candesartan cilexetil (Atacand), eprosartan mesylate (Teveten), irbesartan (Avapro), losartan (Cozaar, Hyzaar), olmesartan (Benicar), telmisartan (Micardis), valsartan (Diovan) | Diarrhea; gastrointestinal problems; muscle cramps; back and leg pain; dizziness; insomnia; nasal congestion; sinus problems; upper respiratory infections |
| **CCBs** | (Formally known as Calcium Channel Blockers). Keeps calcium from entering the cells in the muscles of the blood vessels and heart so they relax more | Generic and corresponding brands: amlodipine (Norvasc), amlodipine and atorvastatin (Caduet), amlodipine and benazepril hydrochloride (Lotrel), diltiazem (Cardizem SR, Dilacor XR, Taztia, Tiazac), enalapril maleate-felodipine ER (Lexxel), felodipine (Plendil), isradipine (DynaCirc), nicardipine (Cardene), nifedipine (Adalat, Procardia XL), nisoldipine (Sular), verapamil (Calan SR, Isoptin SR) | Dizziness; flushing of the face; swelling in the legs from fluid buildup; rapid or slowed heart rate; constipation |
| **ACE inhibitors** | (Formally known as Angiotensin Converting Enzyme inhibitor). Blocks an enzyme that narrows the blood vessels, thus allowing them to relax and widen for smoother blood flow | Generic and corresponding brands: benazepril (Lotensin), captopril (Capoten), enalapril (Vasotec), fosinopril (Monopril), lisinopril (Prinivil, Zestril), perindopril (Aceon), quinapril (Accupril), ramipril (Altace), trandolapril (Mavik) | Dry cough; rash or itching; allergy-like symptoms; allergic reaction with generalized swelling; swelling of the upper airway (in rare cases); excess potassium buildup in the body (especially in people with kidney failure) |
| **Direct renin inhibitors** | Block a certain enzyme from regulating blood pressure (renin), allowing the blood vessels to widen | Generic and corresponding brand: aliskiren (Tekturna) | Diarrhea; rash; allergic reaction that may lead to swelling in the face, lips, tongue or throat (which may make swallowing or breathing difficult) |

Sources: www.webmd.com and www.mayoclinic.com
Chart reviewed by Dr. Joe Brincat, MD

have that are causing the high blood pressure. Many medications are prescribed on a trial-and-error basis. If a mild diuretic doesn't do the trick, then you may be prescribed an alpha blocker. If that doesn't work, then maybe you have too much calcium in the muscle cells, so let's try a calcium channel blocker. If that doesn't work, you may have to move on to the ACE inhibitors and so forth.

## KICKING THE DRUG HABIT: HOW TO FREE YOURSELF FROM HIGH PRICES AND MISERABLE SIDE EFFECTS

Many medications used for the treatment of hypertension play around with heartbeat, blood vessel width, and the reduction of hormones and minerals that impact the blood flow through the vessels. These are imposed conditions that if suddenly changed can cause serious injury to the heart or blood vessels. NEVER STOP TREATMENT WITHOUT CONSULTING YOUR DOCTOR! That cannot be emphasized enough.

Your overall objective is to live a healthier lifestyle, which promotes healthy blood pressure levels. When you decide you want to take a natural approach, the reduction of medication has to be done slowly and under careful doctor supervision. Many doctors will tell you it is risky, but all will surely approve of the natural approach outlined in this book, even if they tell you to couple it with your current regime of medication. Once you have shown your doctor that you are able to eat right, maintain a good weight, exercise regularly, etc., then they are more likely to support your decision to treat hypertension without the use of drugs.

## GETTING YOUR DOCTOR ON YOUR TEAM

If your doctor has approved trying an all-natural approach, you will most likely be carefully and slowly weaned off your current prescriptions. The length of time this takes will depend on a few factors, including age. If you are young, you have more time in the prevention of further strain and damage on the heart that results from years of untreated high blood pressure. Your body can most likely afford to go a little longer with mild hypertension or at a pre-hypertension level before irreversible damage is done.

Older patients with hypertension may be at a higher risk by untreated high blood pressure, since their bodies may have gone through many years of added stress on the heart and blood vessels. However, anyone who wants to make the transition can prove to their doctor they have fully adopted the kind of diet and lifestyle that supports healthy blood pressure readings.

Your transition begins by making the changes outlined in the sixty-day plan while under a doctor's care and instructions for reducing medication. As your body responds to the added exercise, better nutritional balance, and addition of essential minerals, your need for medication can be reduced proportionately.

## CHAPTER SUMMARY

High blood pressure is treatable and prescription drugs are not the only way. Millions of prescriptions are written each year in an effort to lower blood pressure. The reason there are so many types and brands of medication is that no one prescription seems to be able to do the job.

The side effects from hypertension medication may feel worse than the condition. Imagine feeling fine, but being told you have high blood pressure. You are put on a medication that makes you nauseated and dizzy. Then imagine you must take a medication to treat the nausea and dizziness and live with this for the rest of your life. It is enough to make anyone want to try a more natural, healthy approach.

The next chapter addresses what types of vitamins and minerals your body needs to maintain a healthy blood pressure and what levels are needed for achieving your goal of lowering your blood pressure. You will also learn about the use of supplements and how they complement, not replace, dietary nutrients.

# 3

# My Handpicked Essential Vitamins, Minerals, and Herbs That Pass the "Mangano Quality Test"

Everyone knows that you need certain vitamins and minerals to be healthy. Many people are also aware of the fact that much of the food choices in the average American diet fall far short of the recommended amounts of these nutrients.

The Food and Drug Administration (FDA) has set up guidelines known as recommended daily allowances (RDA) that are written in terms of grams (g), milligrams (mg), or micrograms (mcg) on food and supplement packaging. There are also daily values (DV) that are written as percentages on these labels representing how much of the nutrient this particular food gives us out of the total, 100 percent, we should be getting each day.

What you may not be aware of is that there are specific minerals that doctors, scientists, and nutritionists have discovered are beneficial in the management of high blood pressure. Three specific minerals are potassium, calcium, and magnesium.

## THE POWER OF POTASSIUM

Of the three key minerals known to have a positive effect on blood pressure, potassium is the most substantiated. Hundreds, if not thousands, of studies have been conducted in the last few decades, and all confirm that higher levels of potassium lower blood pressure.

One such study was presented at the American Society of Nephrology's 41st Annual Meeting in November of 2008. Researchers from the University of Texas Southwestern Medical Center showed how the amount of potassium found in urine samples was strongly related to whether or not participants had high or low blood pressure levels. Just as sodium is excreted through the urine, so is potassium, and the researchers found in their analysis that participants whose urine samples contained high amounts of potassium tended to have low blood pressure readings. Those with low amounts of potassium had high blood pressure readings. This is the most recent example of a study that confirms the power of potassium.

Generally, when a blood pressure medication or combination of medications is prescribed, doctors expect blood pressure to be lowered by about eight points for systolic readings and about five points for diastolic readings.

A study completed in 1996 by Johns Hopkins Medicine found that potassium supplements were able to accomplish at least half as much of a reduction in blood pressure readings as prescription medications.

For those with a healthy blood pressure, the readings were 3.1 mmHg systolic and 2.0 mmHg diastolic lower when potassium was increased. For those with hypertension, it was even more dramatic. The systolic pressure was reduced by 4.4 mmHg and 2.5 mmHg for diastolic pressure.

A Duke University study came up with even better results. The results of their study showed people dropping their blood pressure by as much as twenty points after just two months of taking potassium supplements.

The same study determined that potassium had even more of an impact on two groups considered to be a higher risk for hypertension. The groups were people with a high salt intake and African-Americans. Both benefited even more from higher levels of potassium.

A leader in this study, Lawrence Appel, M.D., concluded by saying that, "by combining the results of over thirty studies that together enrolled more than

2,500 persons, we conclusively demonstrated that potassium can reduce blood pressure. While this research evaluates potassium in the form of pills or supplements, it is likely, and preferable, that similar benefits would occur from potassium-rich foods."

**Some Potassium Rich Foods**

| Food | Serving Size | Potassium (mg) |
|---|---|---|
| Apricots, dried | 10 halves | 407 |
| Bananas, raw | 1 cup | 594 |
| Beets, cooked | 1 cup | 519 |
| Brussels sprouts, cooked | 1 cup | 504 |
| Cantaloupe | 1 cup | 494 |
| Lima beans | 1 cup | 955 |
| Orange juice | 1 cup | 496 |
| Potatoes, baked, flesh and skin | 1 potato | 1081 |
| Raisins | 1 cup | 1089 |
| Spinach, cooked | 1 cup | 839 |
| Tomato products, canned, sauce | 1 cup | 909 |
| Winter squash | 1 cup | 896 |
| Yogurt, plain, skim milk | 8 oz | 579 |

Source: NHLBI

There is no recommended daily allowance for potassium. However, experts recommend 3,500 mg for an individual with high blood pressure. The average American diet has about 2,500 mg of potassium. In order to get more potassium, you should evaluate and alter your food choices. Using a supplement for potassium should only be done under the direction of your doctor. In addition to the fruits, vegetables, and dairy products listed below, just about any kind of fish can provide a significant amount of potassium to your diet. As you can see there are clearly many ways to safely increase your intake of potassium.

Another word of caution on the use of potassium supplements—it may appear that if you are currently taking a medication, such as those in the diuretic category, that you could be losing potassium and therefore could benefit from adding potassium to your diet with different food choices or a supplement. While some diuretics reduce potassium, others are designed to hold onto potassium. The same is true of some of the medications categorized as ACE inhibitors.

You should consult with your doctor before taking a potassium supplement, especially if you have kidney problems. If your goal is to increase potassium enough that you may not need the medication, you could actually be overdosing on potassium if your current medication is one that causes you to store potassium, instead of the kind that depletes the body of the mineral.

## A Lesson About Lecithin

Another type of supplement that helps you get your potassium and calcium is lecithin. Since lecithin is considered an acquired taste, you can use it in granule form to add to cereal, yogurt, juice or milk. If you are drinking it, you will want to stir it well and drink it quickly, as the granules do not dissolve in cold fluids.

Lecithin granules are comprised of: 90 mg potassium, 56 mg calcium, and 240 mg phosphorus per 7.5 gram serving. This amazing substance is derived from soybeans and is also sometimes considered one of the B-complex vitamins due to the fact that it's a natural source of choline and helps strengthen nerve sheaths. It can also help improve energy levels. Studies have shown that not only can it help reduce cholesterol levels, but it can aid in weight loss as well. Definitely look toward adding lecithin to your daily routine, as it has many healthy benefits in the long run.

## Calcium

Calcium benefits the body in so many ways. We know that it helps build strong teeth and bones. Having strong teeth means fewer cavities, and having strong bones helps prevent certain diseases such as osteoporosis.

What you may not know is that calcium can also reduce blood pressure. The evidence is not as strong or widely accepted by all in the medical profession regarding calcium and the reduction of blood pressure. However, all are in agreement that there is at least some benefit, and that the other health benefits of calcium make it an important mineral in maintaining good health.

The *Journal of the American Medical Association* (JAMA; Apr 3, 1996) published a report on the effectiveness of calcium in reducing high blood pressure. The report emphasizes that calcium has a greater effect on lowering systolic pressure and little effect on diastolic. This is important to note because many people with hypertension may only have a problem with one of the readings depending on which way the blood vessels are being strained—as the heart pumps or in the resting pressure between beats.

One point the studies on calcium do agree upon is that insufficient calcium intake is associated with high blood pressure. So if you are already getting enough calcium in your diet and still have hypertension, more may not help. Or in other words, if your calcium consumption is not adequate, then bringing it up to the proper level can help stabilize your blood pressure.

Lawrence Resnick, M.D., of the Cardiovascular Center at New York Hospital-Cornell Medical Center discovered that adding 2,000 mg of calcium each day counteracted the effect of salt in raising blood pressure. For those who are salt sensitive or just can't seem to cut it from their diet, this is an important finding. If you fall into this category, then calcium may play a much bigger role in reducing your blood pressure.

Supplements can help you get the calcium your diet may lack. They are especially effective if combined with vitamins D and K, which help the body to absorb the calcium. Be cautioned, though. You may think you are getting plenty of calcium, but if your caffeine intake is also high, you could be canceling out the benefits of calcium-rich foods.

The NHLBI cautions that you should choose low fat or nonfat sources of calcium. They actually contain more calcium per serving than the high fat options.

In addition to the calcium-rich foods below, some nondairy sources of calcium include almonds, brussels sprouts, sesame seeds, turnip greens, peas and white beans.

**Some Calcium-Rich Foods**

| Food | Serving Size | Calcium (mg) |
|---|---|---|
| Broccoli, raw | 1 cup | 42 |
| Cheese, cheddar | 1 oz | 204 |
| Milk, fat free or skim | 1 cup | 301 |
| Salmon | 3 oz | 116 |
| Spinach, cooked | 1 cup | 245 |
| Tofu, soft | 1 piece | 133 |
| Yogurt plain, skim milk | 8 oz | 452 |

Source: NHLBI

## MAGNIFICENT MAGNESIUM

Magnesium falls into that inconclusive category like calcium. It has many healthy benefits, but is only effective for some in the treatment of hypertension. It is still recommended that adults get at least 500 mg of magnesium each day because, like calcium a lack of magnesium can elevate blood pressure, even if more magnesium doesn't necessarily lower it.

Magnesium is easy to get in a balanced, traditional American diet. Whole grains are a great source. If you are eating only white bread, a simple change to whole wheat bread may get you all the magnesium you need. In addition, calcium supplements often combine magnesium to help in absorption.

If you are currently taking a high blood pressure medication in the diuretic category, chances are good that it is also depleting your potassium and magnesium. This is why a supplement or extra care in food choices to bring back the 500 mg per day is extremely important. Even if you can remove the medication with your doctor's care, you may need to restore magnesium levels through diet or supplements that provide 400 to 800 mg of magnesium each day.

**Some Magnesium-Rich Foods**

| Food | Serving Size | Magnesium (mg) |
|------|--------------|----------------|
| Beans, black | 1 cup | 120 |
| Halibut | 1/2 fillet | 170 |
| Nuts, peanuts | 1 oz | 64 |
| Seeds, pumpkin, and squash | 1 oz (142 seeds) | 151 |
| Spinach, cooked | 1 cup | 157 |
| Whole grain cereal, cooked | 1 cup | 56 |
| Whole wheat bread | 1 slice | 24 |

Source: NHLBI

## KEEN FOR QUINOA

Another food that's high in magnesium is quinoa. But before I get into just how much magnesium is in quinoa, allow me to explain just what quinoa is. Quinoa (pronounced "keen-wah") is a whole grain seed that has a kernel-like exterior and bears some resemblance to couscous. While quinoa is great to eat at all times of the day, it's frequently used at dinner time in place of side dishes like rice. But unlike rice, quinoa is high in protein. What's more, it's a complete protein, meaning it contains all nine of the essential amino acids—a very uncommon thing for a primarily carbohydrate-based food.

The health benefits of this superfood run the gamut, with studies indicating it can help alleviate migraine symptoms, while others show people who eat foods like quinoa are at a decreased risk for being diagnosed with type II diabetes. And in both cases, magnesium was fingered as the catalyst for such propitious health findings. In just a quarter of a cup, quinoa has about 90 milligrams of magnesium!

And when it comes to treating hypertension, few foods compare to quinoa in effectiveness. According to the Journal of Japanese Society of Nutrition and Food Science, quinoa may help to lower blood pressure rates in those who are hypertensive. Researchers discovered this after feeding quinoa to several groups of hypertensive rats over a six-week period. At the conclusion of their study, they found significant differences in the systolic blood pressure rates of the quinoa-eating groups. The researchers found that the quinoa-eating rats' systolic blood pressure rates were suppressed after just five weeks of regular quinoa feedings, "suggesting that quinoa had a hypotensive effect (meaning a lowering of blood pressure)." The same could not be said for the control group.

While other nutritional composition factors played a role in quinoa's hypotensive qualities—like its richness in potassium and iron—its richness in magnesium played a crucial role, as magnesium naturally relaxes the blood vessels.

## SENSIBLE SUPPLEMENTS

Just a word of caution at the beginning of this section on taking supplements: If a little calcium and magnesium is good, then more must be better, right? WRONG! You can overdose on a good thing as much as a bad thing. It is important to remember that nutrition and health have so much to do with balance. When that balance is thrown off in one direction or another, poor health can result. There are recommended amounts of each nutrient discussed in this book. To go overboard not only wastes your money, it can hurt your health.

There are several other vitamins and minerals in the form of supplements that are believed to help control blood pressure. These include vitamins C and E, omega-3 fatty acids, and coenzyme Q10.

## VITAL VITAMINS: C AND E

A diet and supplement regime that gives you one to three grams of vitamin C a day is thought to be beneficial to maintaining good blood pressure levels. A study conducted by Joseph A. Vita, M.D., who is also an associate professor of medicine at the Boston University School of Medicine, suggested that vitamin C could help dilate blood vessels, thereby lowering blood pressure. After a thirty-day trial, those patients who received two grams of vitamin C had a lower systolic blood pressure. The conclusion drawn by the study was that the higher the vitamin C, the lower the blood pressure (although it was not tested for a longer period of time, so the results could be swayed).

Vitamin C is also generally known to be safe and without side effects.

Vitamin E, on the other hand, may not be as good at managing blood pressure as other vitamins and minerals, but it plays an important role in heart health. Vitamin E is what is known as an antioxidant, which fights potentially toxic free radicals in the body. The free radicals contribute to disease, and the antioxidants—such as those from vitamin E—help protect the body.

As far as controlling blood pressure, vitamin E has more of a role in reversing the degenerative process because of its antioxidant properties. That alone is thought to contribute to the reduction of blood pressure.

So if vitamin C helps to lower blood pressure and vitamin E plays a crucial role in heart health, what about the letter that separates C and E? Does vitamin D have any role to play in the lowering of blood pressure rates?

Vitamin D has received more attention than any other vitamin in the world of health news in recent years, largely stemming from the deficiencies in vitamin D levels doctors are seeing in both children and adults. Perhaps the most well-known of symptoms associated with vitamin D deficiency is improper bone development. Rickets is one such indicator of improper bone development. But more and more health risks outside of rickets are being associated with vitamin D deficiency. For instance, as reported in The Journal of Clinical Endocrinology & Metabolism, pregnant women deficient in vitamin D have a greater likelihood of needing a Cesarean section for birth. Researchers believe this is likely due to poor muscle and bone development during pregnancy, but it may also have something to do with the high blood pressure rates women in need of a C-section tend to have.

The correlation between low vitamin D levels and high blood pressure isn't relegated to this study, mind you. Several studies make similar conclusions. Published in the American Journal of Hypertension, a survey found that people whose vitamin D levels were lowest had the highest blood pressure readings. The study involved approximately 12,600 men and women of all ages (20 and older) and took into account possible contributing factors, like age, gender, ethnicity and physical activity.

So, while vitamin E has a more indirect role in controlling blood pressure due to its antioxidant properties, the roles of vitamins C and D are more direct, in that high vitamin C levels tend to cause a lowering of blood pressure, while low vitamin D levels are linked to high blood pressure readings (it's not yet known if increasing vitamin D levels lowers blood pressure).

## HOW NATURE MADE IT: NATURAL VITAMIN E VS. SYNTHETIC

Natural is always better. We see it in the choice of whole grains versus refined. Why strip the grain, or your diet for that matter, of a nutrient only to add back a synthetic version? It just doesn't make good health sense. You also can't say enough good things about vitamin E. It has been recommended in the prevention of more than eighty different diseases and conditions, not the least of which is hypertension. As an antioxidant, it is one of the best. The right amounts of vitamin E will not only make you feel better, but also look better with clear, smooth skin and shiny hair.

The natural versus synthetic debate is especially true when it comes to vitamin E. Natural sources are better than supplemental sources, and here is why: The body is much more able to process the natural vitamin E than the synthetic, which means that the natural vitamin E is available when the body needs it. In taking synthetic vitamin E, you are only getting 67 percent of what you would get from the same amount in a natural form.

Vitamin E is found in many different foods. These include dark, leafy vegetables, legumes, and nuts. Eggs and soybeans are also good sources, as are wheat germ and brown rice.

Even if you don't eat enough of these foods, you can still get natural vitamin E in the form of a supplement. The label will tell you if you are getting the natural form (d-alpha-tocopherol) or the synthetic form (dl-alpha-tocopherol). The only difference on the label will be the *l* at the beginning, next to the *d.* You will pay a bit more for the natural vitamin E supplement, but you also get one-third more potency and benefit.

With any kind of vitamin E supplement, you need to be careful how and when you take it. If you take a multivitamin with iron or separate iron supplement, the absorption of the vitamin E will be diminished. The two should be taken at different times of the day.

## THE SKINNY ON OMEGA-3 FATTY ACIDS (FISH OILS)

If you eat at least two servings of fish every week, then you probably don't need to supplement your diet with fish oil supplements—those that provide the essential omega-3 fatty acids. You may find that the mercury levels from fish consumption in your body are high, though, and that comes with dangers of its own.

To get the omega-3 fatty acids and, more specifically, the eicosapentaenoic acid (EPA) and docosahexaenoic acid (DHA) into your diet, a supplement is more realistic. The American Heart Association recommends also eating forms of soy that contain alpha-linolenic acid (LNA), which turns to omega-3 fatty acid in the body.

An intake of EPA and DHA has been shown to promote a healthy heart in basically healthy people with a risk of heart disease or high blood pressure. If you are in the pre-hypertension stage, then you may be able to benefit from this the most. So while omega-3 fatty acids only lower blood pressure slightly, they can play a significant role in preventing or postponing higher levels of blood pressure and the resulting heart disease.

## COENZYME Q10: WHAT ONE-THIRD OF HYPERTENSION PATIENTS LACK

Coenzyme Q10 is naturally produced by the body and helps with maintaining metabolic rates. It is recommended that 50 mg of coenzyme Q10 be taken twice a day with food for the best absorption and to minimize upset stomach.

In studies done on people with hypertension, one-third were found to be lacking this important enzyme. Based on a 1994 study, WholeHealthMD.com reports that one-half of the people with hypertension given adequate amounts of coenzyme Q10 were able to go off of one to three of their current blood pressure medications.

If we lived in a perfect world where all of the soils producing our vegetables were not depleted of nutrients, or if we ate our foods in their most whole, raw form, then diet alone would be enough. Unfortunately, most of us like our vegetables cooked, sometimes even prepared quickly in a microwave, and that literally zaps the enzymes from the foods. That is why a supplement is usually the best source of coenzyme Q10 as well as other vitamins.

## SUPERCHARGE YOUR EFFORTS WITH COENZYME A

You've no doubt heard of coenzyme Q10, but what about coenzyme A? This is a lesser-known enzyme with huge benefits to those needing to control their blood pressure.

Enzymes are manufactured at the cellular level and therefore treat and nourish the body at the cellular level. They are the activators of processes and reactions, and work with vitamins. Eating the freshest and most whole forms of foods is the way to ensure maximum benefit from enzymes.

Coenzyme A is made from the cells using vitamin B5, also known as pantothenic acid, and plays a primary role in metabolism. A deficiency of coenzyme A can result in low energy. It can also do some real behind-the-scenes damage to the adrenal gland function, further reducing energy levels.

To ensure you are getting enough of this important enzyme, you probably need to also use a nutritional supplement. The supplement itself does not produce coenzyme A, only the cells in the body can do that. The supplements you take, or foods you need to eat to support the manufacturing process is what's found in bottles at the health store that boast the label "Coenzyme A." These food supplements may be herbs, rich in vitamin B5, or can be taken as capsules or powders. The supplements to support production of coenzyme A contain such ingredients as pantethine acid (vitamin B5), calcium, magnesium, and acetyl L-carnitine.

There are some good food sources from which to get your pantethine acid. These include beans (other than green beans), peas, and other fresh vegetables. You can also get B5 from fish, lean meat, and whole grains. Supplementing with a vitamin supplement is okay for ensuring you measure up in your vitamin B5 consumption, but the food sources are best for having the most energy. It is also good to note that B5 is not lost in cooking as much as with many other vitamins and minerals.

## CLEANING UP WITH BETA GLUCAN

The primary purpose of beta glucan is to boost the immune system. That alone makes it a valuable supplement. By now you've learned that a strong immune system is important in heart health as well. The active components of beta glucan can draw away plaque from the artery walls and allow blood to flow with less pressure on the arteries. In addition, beta glucan removes toxins from the bloodstream by activating the macrophages, which are the immune cells.

Oat bran is probably the best source of beta glucan. It has the ability to naturally lower cholesterol, which is a precursor to other heart-related diseases and conditions. It is easy to get oat bran in the diet through cereals or breads. Just 200 mg of oat bran each day has healthy benefits and works to boost the immune system. Perhaps our great-grandparents knew what they were doing when they served up a hot bowl of oatmeal each morning.

The FDA has not set dietary guidelines of recommended quantities for beta glucan. However, the manufacturers of oat products are allowed by FDA rules to claim that their cereals and breads lower cholesterol and promote a healthy heart.

## MAKING SENSE OF SELENIUM

Selenium is an extremely important mineral in the battle against hypertension. The findings of several studies within the medical and nutritional science fields concluded that insufficient amounts of selenium have been seen in people with certain types of cancers and heart disease. In other words, people with these conditions usually have low levels of this trace mineral. This research can't quite lead to the correlation that low selenium levels cause these conditions, but it is an interesting fact that there is one common denominator.

On the other side of the coin is what nutritionists know with certainty about selenium. Selenium is a trace mineral in the same category as zinc and copper. Selenium, along with zinc and copper, works toward regulating hypertension in a secondary role. Their impact on their own is not significant, but a disproportionate amount of copper to zinc is found in most people with high blood pressure. Too much copper matched to the level of zinc is evident in hypertension patients. So it is with selenium. There is a secondary role in its influence upon hypertension. The proper amounts of selenium in relationship to other minerals can also ward off some cancers, heart disease, and control hypertension.

Selenium works best when it is partnered with vitamin E. Together, the two create a powerful antioxidant that prevents free radicals from forming and weakening the immune system. Other discussions in this book on antioxidants pertain here as well. Antioxidants reverse the degenerative process and boost the immune system, thereby lowering blood pressure naturally.

Whole grains are the best source of selenium. The mineral is only part of the food chemistry because there is selenium in the soil in which the food is grown. This causes a big problem when you are trying to determine just how much selenium is actually in the food. Soils that grow large quantities of commercially sold grains are almost always depleted of minerals.

If you were to grow your own grains and know that the crops were rotated after so many growing seasons to not deplete the soil's minerals, you'd be all set. However, since that is not realistic for most people, then a selenium supplement coupled with vitamin E in both synthetic and natural forms is the most reasonable solution. The recommended dosage of selenium is 200 mcg per day.

## BONE UP ON BIOFLAVONOIDS

Working closely with vitamin C are bioflavonoids. These nutrients in the vitamin category are essential to the absorption of vitamin C. Bioflavonoids, sometimes called the "P" vitamins keep vitamin C from breaking down before the body can metabolize it.

There are different types of bioflavonoids that you will see on vitamin C supplements. Different categories have different health benefits, but all are believed to work as an antioxidant in preventing free radical damage and in the strengthening of the capillaries, those tiniest of blood vessels.

Bioflavonoids increase circulation. This effect is why it is a valuable supplement for those with hypertension. Less pressure on the blood vessels by way of increased ease of circulation is one way to reduce blood pressure.

Citrus fruits are some of the best sources of natural bioflavonoids. It is actually that white coating on the fruit that comes off with the peel that is the best source. The more that you can keep on and eat with the fruit, the better. Also the pulp and whole fruit provides the most nutrition. Hawthorne berries are also a good source of bioflavonoids and have the added benefit of widening blood vessels, further helping to reduce blood pressure.

## FIGHTING HEART DISEASE WITH FOLIC ACID AND VITAMIN B6

You have probably heard that it is important for pregnant women to get enough folic acid, since deficiencies during pregnancy have been linked to neural tube defects such as spina bifida, a birth defect where the top of the spinal cord is not completely formed. In fact, if all women of childbearing age took folic acid supplements, neural tube defects would be reduced by at least 40 percent.

What you may not realize is that folic acid is just as important in the prevention of heart disease. Folic acid reduces homocysteine in the blood. High levels of homocysteine have been linked to heart disorders and arteriosclerosis. When homocysteine is not countered by folic acid, it turns into an extremely toxic substance. This happens when you try to digest proteins. If there is sufficient folic acid in the diet through foods and supplements, then the homocysteine is converted into a harmless amino acid. Vitamins B6 and B12 aid the folic acid in this process, so the three together are an important combination.

There have been numerous studies conducted on the relationship between elevated levels of homocysteine and high blood pressure. For older people, a 1997 study in *Circulation* indicated that high levels of homocysteine were an independent risk factor in the onset of hypertension. Further studies have concluded that type II diabetes patients with high levels of homocysteine also had high diastolic blood pressure readings. A large-scale study in Norway found that even those with no serious disease but elevated homocysteine levels had high blood pressure as well and were at a higher risk of heart disease.

Even on its own, vitamin B6 can lower blood pressure. A study where twenty patients with hypertension were given 75 mg daily of vitamin B6 for four weeks concluded that the vitamin decreased levels of epinephrine. Epinephrine causes the blood vessels to constrict and makes the heart have to beat harder, putting more force on the arteries and raising blood pressure. By lowering epinephrine, the arteries are able to relax and the blood flows more freely.

While supplementing with vitamin B6 and folic acid are the quickest, easiest way of ensuring a high dose of quality nutrients to help lower blood pressure and keep them low, some may prefer to get their nutrients through food. That's fine, the caveat being the amount of nutrients won't be nearly as high as what's found in a supplement. That being said, the best food sources for vitamin B6 include spinach (.44 mg in one cup), bell peppers (.23 mg in one cup) and turnip greens (.26 mg in one cup). The best protein source is tuna, yielding about 1.20 mg of B6 in a four ounce serving. For folic acid, the best source is a simple bowl of cereal. There are many quality, whole grain cereals that are ultra fortified with folic acid, like oat bran and Kashi's Heart to Heart. And most of them contain the recommended daily value, 400 micrograms, in just three quarters of a cup! But 400 micrograms is the recommended daily value for the average person whose blood pressure levels are normal. For people battling hypertension, they should be consuming twice the daily recommended folic acid levels - about 800 micrograms per day.

## THE L-ARGININE LINK

L-arginine is an amino acid that produces molecules of nitric oxide. It is nitric oxide that has an impact on hypertension. In short, nitric oxide is a vasodilator. In fact, it is one of the most powerful vasodilators that relaxes and stretches the arterial walls, allowing blood to flow more freely, thereby lowering blood pressure. It is also a good antioxidant, helping to maintain a strong immune system.

Naturally, the body releases short bursts of nitric oxide from the lining of the arteries. This keeps the platelets from sticking to the walls, which prevents a build-up that can contribute to hypertension and other heart diseases.

In early experimentation with L-arginine, physicians initially injected the amino acid into patients with hypertension. This quickly and effectively lowered blood pressure. The next step was to introduce an oral option. This, too, proved to work well. An Italian study concluded that just 2 grams of arginine taken orally for one week lowered systolic blood pressure by 20 mmHg.

The right amount of L-arginine in the diet is about 6 grams per day. Ideally, two grams taken three times per day is the way to get it. This is because the reaction is quick and it is better to have the process repeated throughout the day. Animal proteins are the best source of arginine, but eating too much meat isn't good either. The best way to supplement your diet to get enough arginine, then, is with a 500-mg capsule or powder that can be mixed into a beverage. One to two grams taken three times a day is best. Work up to the 2 grams slowly over the course of a couple of weeks. It is also recommended that arginine be taken with food, especially a carbohydrate and preferably without other proteins, since that can negatively impact the absorption.

It is not recommended that people with viral infections take L-arginine supplements or eat foods that contain the amino acid. Nor is it a good idea for pregnant or lactating women to take any L-arginine supplements since it is not clear what the impact could be on the fetus and infant.

In addition to animal proteins, foods containing L-arginine include gelatin, peanuts, soybeans, wheat, and wheat germ. There is also arginine in dairy products, white flour, and chocolate, all of which should be limited because of the lesser nutritional benefits and a greater likelihood of allergic reactions.

## HEART-HEALTHY HERBS

Two herbs generally regarded as heart healthy are garlic and hawthorn. While garlic impacts blood, hawthorn has an effect on the blood vessels.

Garlic works by lowering cholesterol in the blood. Its active ingredient is allicin. This is what slows down the formation of clots, which can clog the arteries with plaque. With less plaque taking up space in the arteries, blood flows through easier and reduces blood pressure.

Hawthorn actually widens the blood vessels. It does this the same way the ACE-inhibitor medications are designed to do it. The hawthorn keeps the angiotensin-converting enzyme (ACE) from constricting the arteries. Hawthorn is also thought to keep the heart muscles strong.

## THE STRENGTHENING POWERS OF GRAPE SEED EXTRACT

There is plenty of good news and research when it comes to the powerful impact of the tiny seeds found in grapes. Actually, grape seed extract in supplement form is usually made from the seeds and sometimes the outer skin of red grapes (Vitis vinifera). The antioxidant capabilities of the grape seed are thought to be even more powerful than both vitamin C and vitamin E. The flavonoids from these grapes are what have had medical researchers of late debating the benefits of red wine in protecting the body against heart disease. It is these same red grapes used to make the wine that provide the beneficial properties. Therefore, juices that use the whole grape and extracts give you all of the benefits of wine without any of the negative aspects of fermentation or risk of possible overconsumption.

Proanthocyanidins, (PCOs) are the most beneficial of the flavonoids found in grape seed extract. They have the ability to strengthen blood vessels and increase circulation. The more flexible the blood vessels are because of added strength allows blood to flow through without added pressure; while the ease of blood circulation reduces the amount of constant pressure on the blood vessels.

In the prevention of heart disease, grape seed extract can keep plaque from forming on the arteries and prevent clots and clogs from developing. Research has indicated that the same anticoagulant effect people get from aspirin therapy is accomplished by grape seed extract, which keeps the blood platelets from sticking together.

Grape seed extract has other health benefits beyond controlling blood pressure. It helps in the management of cholesterol. It can raise HDL, which is the good cholesterol, while it lowers triglyceride levels. Furthermore, grape seed extract has the ability to enter the brain cells and protect them from damage due to free radicals. By penetrating cell membranes, it is a more effective antioxidant.

Treating high blood pressure with grape seed extract is easy. There are no known negative side effects, even after decades of research, with no reported toxic reactions or adverse interactions with other drugs. It can be taken in a tablet, capsule, or liquid form at any time of the day. However, you should be consistent in what time of day you choose to take the supplement and shoot for the same time each day to keep the levels steady in your blood stream.

A daily dose of 100 mg two or three times per day is recommended. The supplement you take should contain standardized grape seed extract containing 92 to 95 percent PCOs.

## THE RIGHT FOOD AND SUPPLEMENT MIX

All this talk about getting enough magnesium and vitamin C, coupled with the necessary intake of selenium and coenzyme A may seem complicated. It can make you feel like you will be forced to pop fifty different supplements three times a day and eating 5,000 calories, which would never allow you to lose weight and stay active. The best way to be sure you are getting everything you need in your diet without overeating or taking dozens of supplements is by making the right choices. The right choices in foods are those that provide several heart-healthy nutrients.

Many foods contain at least four or five of the best nutrients for battling hypertension. You don't need to eat broccoli for the calcium and then potatoes for the magnesium and bison for the protein. You can get all of these nutrients in one whole, organically grown portion of peaches, which contains protein, potassium, and calcium.

The choices you make in your diet should involve getting as much of the nutritional requirements you need in as few food choices as possible. This takes some planning, and hopefully the education about nutrition in this book will help you with your choices as you see the cross-nutritional value of many different foods.

Once you have planned your diet, including foods from different food groups and those known to promote healthy blood pressure, then you look to see where supplements may be needed. Remember, the goal is to get the nutrition from the food. The supplement is a last resort, so to speak. If you choose unhealthy processed foods all the time, then it would take many supplements to put back the nutrients in your diet, and even then, they can't do as good a job as most healthy foods.

In choosing supplements, there are also many that combine vitamins and minerals and antioxidants into formulas that can be effectively used without separate capsules. Reputable manufacturers will also create formulas of vitamins and minerals, which can be blended without negating the effects of another ingredient or reducing their absorption. With some careful planning, you can create a menu of the fewest calories with the best nutrition and limit the number of supplements needed daily.

## DAILY DOSAGES OF BEETROOT JUICE TO BEAT HIGH BLOOD PRESSURE

Did you know that drinking only 500 ml of beetroot juice a day can significantly lower your blood pressure? A study presented in the *American Heart Association Journal* was recently published to support this natural healing alternative. Professors of The London School of Medicine were the key leaders of this study and found proof of the natural healing of beetroot juice.

The study shows that it is the ingestion of the dietary nitrate in the beetroot juice, which can also be found in other leafy vegetables that is ultimately responsible for the lowered blood pressure. From observing different volunteers, the researchers of this study found that blood pressure levels were lowered within only one hour after drinking the beetroot juice. Amazing results!

With this degree of lowered blood pressure observed from one day of drinking this juice, imagine the results of drinking 500 ml of it each day for a year!

With hypertension causing around 50 percent of coronary heart disease, it is important to find these natural solutions to help lower your high blood pressure before it leads to more serious and life threatening avenues.

Beetroot juice is available to purchase, although it may not be as readily available as supplements. You can also make your own fresh beetroot juice, which I recommend. It is a very tasty beverage, but remember: more is not necessarily better, so pay close attention and measure your juice carefully before ingestion.

By including the correct amount of beetroot juice in your diet once a day, you are greatly improving your blood pressure with just a little bit of work!

## DARK CHOCOLATE AND YOUR LOWER BLOOD PRESSURE

Before I get started, you should know that, unfortunately, I'm not talking about consuming your favorite chocolate bar from the local grocery store to help lower your high blood pressure! The dark chocolate I'm referring to is the real herbal dark chocolate, otherwise known as raw cacao.

A study published in the *Archives of Internal Medicine* speaks highly of what cacao and cocoa can do for your high blood pressure. This study was organized with the aim to compare the results of cacao versus tea for lowering high blood pressure. With ten studies done in total, five for each method over a period of ten years, cocoa and cacao came out on top.

The consumption of dark chocolate, or raw cacao, was found to lower high blood pressure by 4.7/2.8 mmHg. On the other hand, in the five tea studies, no significant change occurred. This form of dark chocolate offers different properties than tea. While tea is high in flavonoids, dark chocolate such as this is high in procyanidins. It is exactly this property within the dark chocolate that has the potential to lower high blood pressure as well as the number of strokes by 20 percent.

Although this discovery has been found to be effective, I'm not encouraging you to go out and consume large amounts of raw cacao all at once to get instant results. This study was based on only a small square of raw cacao on a daily basis. Remember that there are negative aspects of dark chocolate, even if the cacao content is high because dark chocolates such as this can be high in calories and sugar; use it wisely to avoid gaining weight.

## BOOST YOUR OLIVE OIL INTAKE FOR RESULTS

A new study that recently appeared in an issue of *Journal of Nutrition* stated that the more olive oil men consume in their daily diets, the more they will be able to lower their high blood pressure levels naturally.

In our society today, olive oil is not an ingredient or supplement that is widely used. This study took a group of men and created a study schedule of three, three-week periods of 25 ml of olive oil intake a day, plus supplementation and then two weeks of non-supplementation. This study showed, in the end, that the men's blood pressure levels had dropped 2 to 3 percent after this olive oil supplementation.

In terms of your blood pressure, 2 to 3 percent is a significant drop that can really make a difference in how you feel and in the prevention of further heart diseases such as stroke or coronary heart disease. If you are a man who does not consume olive oil already, then this is a great natural alternative to the prescription medications available for high blood pressure today.

Make sure to consume moderate amounts so as not to alter your weight. There are dozens of healthy recipes that include olive oil in them that you are sure to like, which makes this natural remedy simple to follow and enjoyable as well.

## YOUR CHOICE OF HERBAL SUPPLEMENTS

Let's talk about the different herbs that can help lower your high blood pressure through their own natural and unique properties. This type of awareness can help you avoid the prescription medications that can be so harmfully addictive, and keep you on the natural path to a clean bill of health.

One of the most popular, and perhaps the most obscure of all herbal treatments for high blood pressure, is to take several different herbs and use their healing properties together. You can use herbs such as Indian gooseberry, winter cherry, hundred husbands, muskroot, saffron, and licorice, just to name a few. Each of these herbs has healing properties that can contribute to lowering your blood pressure. Others include:

**Arjuna bark**, which can be found throughout India, has been used for medicinal purposes for more than three centuries, so you can be sure it works! Several studies have shown that it has the ability to lower high blood pressure and even prevent different heart diseases. Prolonged use has no harmful side effects.

**Black cumin seeds** contain an essential oil potent enough to help lower high blood pressure through small dosages. These seeds have a long history of medicinal use through different ages of folk medicine and the same remedies can still be used successfully today.

**Forskolin** is an herb that has been shown to have a positive effect on hypertension by relaxing the arterial vascular smooth muscle.

**Hawthorn** has been used to treat heart disease and high blood pressure for centuries. It has been shown to mildly lower high blood pressure after four weeks of taking it. This herb has the ability to dilate your coronary blood vessels, something not many other herbs can do. Also, even if you are still taking prescription blood pressure medications, it is completely safe to take hawthorn as well.

**Maitake** is a type of mushroom that has been shown to have major effects on cholesterol and high blood pressure over the years. With a recommended dosage of 3 to 7 grams daily, it is a safe and effective way to naturally lower your blood pressure levels.

**European mistletoe** possesses the ability to inhibit hypertension diseases as well as common heart conditions. Many studies have shown and publicized its success and therefore it is readily available anywhere supplements and herbs are sold.

**Olive leaf** can be found on olive trees and contains a complex makeup of substances that act to lower high blood pressure. Studies have shown significant results without side effects.

**Yarrow** contains substances that are able to greatly lower your blood pressure levels with small and consistent dosages. Approximately two months of treatment is recommended.

## NATURAL ALTERNATIVES: HOMEOPATHY

Studies have shown that using any one homeopathic remedy steadily and carefully for only one month will provide you with the results you need to continually lower your high blood pressure the safest way possible. The important aspect to remember about homeopathic remedies is that they can affect everyone differently. If side effects arise, stop treatment immediately and visit a professional naturopathic to help you with your treatments.

Arum is a homeopathic remedy that has been used for centuries to treat a number of different and common ailments, including high blood pressure and heart disease. Arum is a warm and soothing compress that is applied to the chest to help relieve the symptoms from outside the body.

Belladonna was one of the first developed homeopathic remedies for hypertension, and is still one of the most trusted natural alternatives to Western medicine. Belladonna is a plant that is taken and crushed to extract the natural juices and it is the juice that offers the healing properties for hypertension sufferers today.

By choosing one of these successful homeopathic remedies and sticking with it for at least one month, you may find you have lowered your blood pressure levels by at least 3 percent. You can find these homeopathic remedies through many natural alternative health stores and homeopathic retailers today.

## CHAPTER SUMMARY

This chapter has talked mainly about supplementing a diet that is lacking in vitamins, minerals, and other nutrients known to keep blood pressure levels healthy. Dietary supplements are one way, but nothing really is better than a healthy eating plan that incorporates as many of the nutrients as possible in natural form.

The following chart is a summary of the vitamins, minerals, and herbs discussed in this chapter and the recommended amounts of each to lower blood pressure or prevent it from rising.

The next chapter addresses how diet choices, both the good and bad, can greatly impact blood pressure by providing the right nutrients.

**Recommended Amounts of Vitamins, Minerals, and Herbs for Healthy Blood Pressure Levels**

| Substance | Recommended Dosage | Comments |
|---|---|---|
| Potassium | 3,500 mg daily from food sources *only.* Avoid or limit supplement use unless directed by a doctor, especially if you have kidney problems. | Potassium deficiency has been linked to high blood pressure. Low levels may result in heart palpitations. |
| Calcium | 1,000 mg daily for average adult, 2,000 mg/day in blood pressure management | Calcium deficiency has also been linked to high blood pressure. |
| Magnesium | 600 to 1,000 mg daily | Magnesium enhances circulation by allowing the muscles in the arterial walls to rest. Take 100 to 200 mg in the morning on an empty stomach and the rest before bedtime. |
| Selenium | 200 mcg daily | Deficiency has been linked to heart disease. |
| Lecithin granules | 7.5 g daily added to foods or liquid. | Lecithin is derived from soy and supplies the body with inositol, choline, and phosphatidyl choline. All three nutrients help maintain healthy arteries and emulsify fat. |
| Vitamin C | 1,000 mg three times a day | Vitamin C is essential and works to prevent a host of different ailments. It is quickly excreted from the body, so it should be consumed several times per day. |
| Vitamin E | 400 IU (international units)/ daily | Vitamin E is helpful in preventing blood clots, therefore helping to prevent strokes and heart attacks. Look for natural vitamin E. |
| Omega-3 fatty acids (fish oils) | 1,000 mg three times a day | Omega-3 fatty acids help minimize the risk of heart disease and other ailments. |

**Recommended Amounts of Vitamins, Minerals, and Herbs for Healthy Blood Pressure Levels**

| Substance | Recommended Dosage | Comments |
| --- | --- | --- |
| Coenzyme Q10 | 50 mg twice daily | Coenzyme Q10 is a powerful antioxidant that prevents oxidation damage and hardening of the arteries. |
| Coenzyme A | As directed on label | Coenzyme A works with coenzyme Q10 to support immune system detoxification. |
| Garlic | 500 mg twice daily | Garlic plays an important role in lowering blood pressure. |
| Hawthorn | 100 to 150 mg three times a day | Hawthorn widens the blood vessels and is thought to keep heart muscles strong. |
| Bioflavonoids | 100 to 300 mg daily | Bioflavonoids protect against cardiovascular disease. Some excellent food sources include the white membrane in oranges and grapefruits, grapes, plums, apricots, cherries, currants, and blackberries. |
| Folic acid | 800 mcg daily | Folic Acid reduces levels of homocysteine in the blood, a substance linked to heart disorders. Food sources include leafy green vegetables, spinach, romaine lettuce, beans, tomatoes, and citrus fruits. |
| Vitamin B complex | 100 mg daily | Vitamin B Complex plays an important role in circulatory function and in lowering blood pressure. |
| L-Arginine | As directed on label | Simply put, this amino acid enables the muscles in the arterial walls to relax. |

# 4

# Making Your Heart Love You

A diet that helps lower blood pressure is one that is going to favor a healthy heart as well. There is common talk about how "good" and "bad" cholesterol affect your heart, and which foods to avoid or eat in moderation in order to keep the good cholesterol high and the bad cholesterol low. Many of the same food choices will contribute to a blood-pressure-reducing diet as well.

Eating right is so important to good health. We all know how we feel after we've indulged in something high in fat or sugar. It sure tastes good going down, but most often within an hour that good feeling is replaced with lethargy. When it comes to eating right for blood pressure management, we don't always get such immediate signals from our bodies—either good or bad. That is why monitoring blood pressure regularly is so important to knowing if our eating habits are helping or hurting the cause.

Some facts we do know about diet and blood pressure are:

- Maintaining an ideal weight through healthy eating and exercise will lower blood pressure.

- Everyone should be getting five servings of fruits and vegetables EVERY day.

- Choosing fruits and vegetables that are high in potassium and calcium will help regulate blood pressure. (See the food lists in previous chapter.)

- Sodium, the added table salt kind and the kind found in processed food, should be used extremely sparingly.

## TRIM THE FLAB, STAY IN SHAPE, AND FEEL GREAT

One sure way to get control of your blood pressure if you are overweight is to lose the weight. The National Institute of Health indicates that a body mass index (BMI) over 25 indicates you weigh too much for your height. A BMI of 30 or above means you are obese. BMI is measured using a table of weight compared to height. Muscle mass is figured into that because muscle weighs more than fat, therefore a lean, muscular person will have more good weight.

To figure yours out, you can use the following formula from the Center for Disease Control (CDC):

Body Mass Index can be calculated using pounds and inches with this equation:

$$BMI = \left[ \frac{\text{Weight in Pounds}}{(\text{Height in Inches}) \times (\text{Height in Inches})} \right] \times 703$$

For example, a person who weighs 220 pounds and is 6 feet 3 inches tall has a BMI of 27.5. It is figured like this:

$$\frac{220 \text{ lb}}{(75 \text{ inches}) \times (75 \text{ inches})} \times 703 = 27.5$$

The results are interpreted as:

| BMI | Weight Status |
|---|---|
| Below 18.5 | Underweight |
| 18.6 to 24.9 | Normal |
| 25.0 to 29.9 | Overweight |
| 30.0 and above | Obese |

Source: CDC

In order to lose weight, the simple route is to take in fewer calories, or burn more calories through exercise than you take in. A pound of body weight is equal to 3,500 calories. To lose one pound, that means that you need to reduce your caloric intake by 3,500. Of course you could starve yourself for a day or two, and there would go one pound. Since it is ridiculous to think that is the way to lose weight, you must work to reduce your calories a little each day.

A healthy weight loss is one where you lose no more than one to two pounds per week. It is also the best way to make a lifelong change in eating habits that will keep the weight off forever.

Start by looking at what you eat each day. The food choices and the number of calories should be evaluated. Then reduce the calories by 500 per day, which will equal 3,500 per week or a one-pound weight loss per week. The final chapter of this book will get more specific in making food choices high in potassium and low in fat and calories as a winning combination for lowering blood pressure through successful weight loss.

## TAKING THE MYSTERY OUT OF EATING RIGHT

Foods high in potassium are easy to find. The chart in the previous chapter outlines some of them. There are also many other considerations in choosing good foods. When we buy a fresh bunch of spinach, we know that we are getting a nutrient-rich food that will help manage blood pressure. What about a can of spinach? Popeye ate it all the time and look at him!

Unfortunately pre-packaged and canned foods are not always what they appear to be. The good news is that the FDA has made it mandatory for manufacturers to disclose every ingredient in a package and other nutritional facts, so READ THE LABELS!

It is so important that you know exactly what is going into your body if you want to effectively manage your blood pressure through diet. A can of spinach can be processed with so much sodium used to preserve and flavor it that you would be better off not eating the spinach at all.

Here is a sample food label to help illustrate this point. It is from a low-calorie, low-carbohydrate frozen dinner, which has the following nutritional analysis on its label:

| | |
|---|---|
| **Calories** | 230 |
| **Total Fat** | 9 g (13%) |
| **Cholesterol** | 55 mg (19%) |
| **Sodium** | 750 mg (31%) |
| **Total Carbohydrates** | 1 g (4%) |
| **Dietary Fiber** | 3 g (11%) |

The percentages are the Recommended Daily Allowances (RDA) based on a 2,000-calorie diet.

Now let's look at the RDAs for an average diet of 2,000 calories versus a diet of 2,500 calories. The chart on food labels states that your caloric intake may need to be lower or higher. This depends on your personal activity level and your age.

**Recommended Daily Allowances**

| Calories | | 2,000 | 2,500 |
|---|---|---|---|
| Total Fat | Less than | 65 g | 80 g |
| Saturated Fat | Less than | 20 g | 25 g |
| Cholesterol | Less than | 300 mg | 300 mg |
| Sodium | Less than | 2,400 mg | 2,400 mg |
| Total Carbohydrates | Average | 300 g | 375 g |
| Dietary Fiber | Average | 25g | 30g |

Now, if you were to make a meal from scratch that is approximately the same portion size as the frozen dinner sample above—using only fresh food, including lean beef, snap peas, water chestnuts, and mushrooms—here is the breakdown:

| | |
|---|---|
| **Calories** | 207 |
| **Total fat** | 8 g (12%) |
| **Cholesterol** | 40 g (11%) |
| **Sodium** | 57 mg (2%) |
| **Total Carbohydrates** | 8 g (3%) |

It is easy to compare and see that the processed and packaged foods contain much more sodium, cholesterol, and carbohydrates, and often more fat, although this case was minimal, because it was a frozen "diet" entrée.

## TIPS TO HELP WITH FAT LOSS, HIGH BLOOD PRESSURE, AND JOINT PAIN

Besides being aware of RDAs and the nutritional content of foods, there are several other beneficial things you should know:

### *Essential Fatty Acids*

Essential fatty acids (EFAs) are specific fatty acids that are necessary for the body to stay healthy. There are three main types of EFAs. These are commonly known as omega-3 (linolenic acid), omega-6 (linoleic acid), and omega-9 (oleic acid). They are also known as healthy fats or good fats. The body needs these EFAs to help it break down and attack bad fats and to even repair some of the damage done by bad fats. Research has shown that essential fatty acids can help with fat loss, can help to lower blood pressure, and can help decrease joint pain.

Essential fatty acids cannot be synthesized by the body, but instead must be obtained through diet. Essential fatty acids can be found in some foods, specifically many types of fish. They are also found in flaxseed oil, grape seed oil, and canola oil. However, the easiest and most reliable way to get EFAs is through a dietary supplement.

A study done by Northwestern University in Chicago revealed that a diet rich in omega-3 fatty acids can help lower blood pressure. The study involved 4,680 men and women living in the United States, Britain, China, and Japan.

Omega-3 fatty acids are beneficial for reducing joint pain and inflammation according to Dr. Jacob Teitelbaum in his book, *Pain Free 1-2-3*. He states that over the last several hundred years, the typical diet has had less and less intake of EFAs. This can be corrected through diet as well as through supplements.

## Exercise

Exercise plays an important role in helping achieve weight loss, control high blood pressure, and alleviate joint pain. Exercise burns many more calories than the body burns in a resting state. In order to produce weight loss, the body needs to exercise to use up excess calories. Exercising also helps the body establish a higher metabolism rate, making it easier to burn calories.

Exercise can also help control and lower high blood pressure. Research has shown that even minimal daily exercise can help control high blood pressure without medication. The body requires some exercise to keep it functioning at its best.

A study published in the *Journal of Epidemiology and Community Health* found that thirty minutes of moderate exercise, three times a week helped lower blood pressure of the participants considerably. The participants were all inactive when they started the study, but were introduced to an exercise regime for twelve weeks. This finding shows that even minimal amounts of regular exercise play a keen role in lowering blood pressure.

Exercise is also an important factor in reducing joint pain. Keeping joints moving helps keep them limber. People who limited their use of certain joints due to pain actually caused the joints to tighten and harden even further, making movement more painful. The solution is to use exercise specific to the type of joint pain you have. Keep the exercises easy and don't overdo the amount. The idea is to keep the joints moving to reduce the amount of pain you have.

A recent study published in the journal *Arthritis Research Therapy* found that exercise can help reduce, and in some cases even prevent, the joint pain often associated with arthritis. The study targeted those with arthritis and added just small amounts of exercise each week. Those who exercised about an hour and fifteen minutes each week reduced the chances of developing pain symptoms by 28 percent. The same study found that more exercise per week (two and a half hours per week) reduced the actual pain symptoms—not just the *chances* of developing pain symptoms—by as much as 46 percent.

### *Reishi Mushroom*

The Reishi mushroom is an ancient Eastern medicine that has been used for hundreds of years. The healing and medicinal properties of the Reishi mushroom are almost endless. It offers help for those with high blood pressure, those who need to lose weight, and those with joint pain. The best part is that the treatment is natural with few, if any, side effects.

Experts have found that the Reishi mushroom offers protection against heart disease and can lower blood pressure. The Reishi lowers triglyceride levels, removes excess cholesterol from the blood, and lowers overall blood pressure. A study reported by Burton Goldberg in *The Definitive Guide To Heart Disease* found that patients who had hypertension and were unresponsive to traditional medications were able to lower their blood pressure significantly by taking Reishi extract three times a day for just four weeks.

Taking Reishi can also help you lose weight. The Reishi has diuretic properties that help the body eliminate water more easily and prevent excess water from being stored. While helping to eliminate water, it also provides energy and maintains balance and focus, which helps those on a diet.

The Reishi mushroom is a powerful pain reliever for those with joint pain and arthritis as well. Research done by Dr. William B. Stavinhoa of the University of Texas Health Science Center has shown that the pain relieving effects of Reishi were as strong as five milligrams of hydrocortisone, but with fewer, if any, side effects.

The Reishi mushroom is strictly used for medicinal purposes rather than for consumption. The mushroom itself is rather hard and woody and has a bitter taste. It is comprised of about 90 percent indigestible fiber. It is therefore most often found in capsule, tablet, or extract form. Taking vitamin C with Reishi may also boost its medicinal powers.

## THE MANGANO VIEW ON MEAT

Not all meat is created equally; neither is all protein. Many people, when they think of getting protein in their diet, automatically assume it needs to come from meat or that meat is the best source. The truth is that there are many great sources of protein and some of them are meats.

For the purpose of discussion, this section will lump together all animal proteins in one category of meat. This includes chicken, turkey, other poultry, wild game, beef, pork, and fish. In choosing any meat from this group, the number one consideration for optimal heart health is choosing the leanest meats possible. This starts out with most varieties of fish, then turkey, skinless chicken breast, and then lean cuts of beef. There is, however, another source of very lean, high protein meat that is not common in the American diet, but is relatively accessible from meat distributors—bison.

Bison, more commonly known as buffalo, are strictly vegetarians. Their diet of grasses makes their meat nutritious and lean. "Lean" and "nutritious" are words frequently associated with skinless chicken breast. Surprisingly the nutritional profile of bison meat leaves the traditional chicken breast looking like a nutritional lightweight (or should I say featherweight?). For example, roasted bison meat has 60 percent more calcium, 350 percent more zinc and a whopping 500 percent more iron than a similarly sized piece of chicken. The same goes for calorie content. A 4 ounce piece of bison meat has 18 fewer calories than a 4 ounce skinless chicken breast (about 178 calories to 160 calories). For fat, chicken and bison are comparable, both yielding a measly 2 grams of fat per four ounce piece (2.2 grams of fat for bison, 2.3 grams of fat for a skinless chicken breast).

If the idea of eating buffalo or bison does not appeal to you, consider using this healthy meat in recipes instead of as a filet-type serving. Any butcher can grind the meat, so it can be used in any recipe that calls for ground beef. The same is true of ground turkey. Once seasoning for recipes like chili or a casserole is added, you will not even be able to tell another meat has been substituted for ground beef.

Just as not all meats are created equally, not all animals are treated equally, or humanely for that matter. If you find you are not quite at the level of being a vegetarian, but have issues with meat production, you can choose only freerange chicken, pork, or other poultry. Moral issues aside, these animals provide healthier alternatives to caged animals. Animals held in close confinement are stressed. This impacts the kinds of chemicals they produce as part of their natural survival instincts.

Meat producers go one step further in creating meats that are plumper and meatier and provide larger cuts. To do this, animals are injected with hormones that increase growth. Chickens can also be fooled into laying more eggs than they naturally would. All of these "enhancements" provide great profits to the meat manufacturers, but compromise the nutritious value and can create harmful side effects. The hormones that are put into the animals are passed on to the meat we eat. The result of eating too much hormone-laden meat leads to such things as early onset of menses in young girls or the development of breasts in boys.

The important things to remember about meat are the following:

1. Eat lean cuts in moderation. Many restaurants sell 16-ounce portions; a healthy portion is about 4 to 6 ounces.

2. Choose meats that are organic, meaning they have not been raised with hormones or chemicals.

3. Choose free-range meats. These animals have not been caged and provide healthier food.

4. Substitute fatty meats with leaner options in recipes. Almost any meat can be ground and used in recipes calling for ground beef.

5. Always remove the skin from chicken and other poultry before cooking to remove most of its fat.

## WHERE SODIUM BELONGS IN YOUR DIET: THE ANSWER WILL SURPRISE YOU

You will probably be surprised that there is something good said about sodium in a book about naturally managing your blood pressure. True, your doctor may have told you to limit the amount of salt you add to your food and even to watch out for hidden sources found in pre-packaged foods and certain condiments such as soy sauce and Worcestershire sauce. This is certainly good advice. It is unrefined sea salt, which is calcium and magnesium naturally blended together, that plays a role in the management of blood pressure by working in harmony with potassium. Even those with hypertension can have some unrefined sea salt when it is balanced with other minerals. Too much can throw off the balance between sodium and potassium and disrupt the electrical system of the body, but an amount of about 2,400 mg per day is generally safe. That recommended amount increases if you are more active and get plenty of exercise.

It is recommended that your daily sodium intake be less than 2,400 mg a day if your blood pressure is normal. If you have hypertension, most doctors will recommend reducing that further. Just as a comparison, a teaspoon of table salt contains about the same amount of sodium as your full daily allowance. You may think that because you never add salt to your foods, you are okay, but just look at the label we previewed before. This one, low-calorie part of a meal contains one-third of the sodium for the entire day. And that is for a person with healthy blood pressure!

The lesson to be learned here is that sodium is hidden in packaged foods and in higher quantities than you may be aware of. Read the labels. Choose fresh, whole, unprocessed foods whenever possible. Anything that is canned or commercially frozen is designed to last a long time on your shelf or in your home freezer. To do this, additives and preservatives—usually some form of sodium—are included.

To help understand how this all works, it is important to understand how sodium works. Sodium is found throughout the body. Two-thirds of it enters the body from the small intestine into the blood and the remaining one-third goes into the bones. All of the sodium the body gets is through food and water. It is excreted through sweat and urine and the excess is stored in tissues of the muscles and cartilage. The kidneys are responsible for regulating the sodium as directed by the pituitary gland, which secretes the hormone aldosterone. Aldosterone either signals the kidneys to put some sodium into the bloodstream or get rid of it when there is enough. All other minerals, such as potassium and calcium, are impacted by sodium and vice versa.

Sodium in the body has four key purposes:

- Regulation of the heartbeat

- Control of nerve impulses and muscle contraction

- Conversion of glucose to glycogen

- Keeping other minerals in proportion

Some other functions of sodium include balancing fluids in body tissues and maintaining pH balance.

High sodium is dangerous when it is disproportional to other minerals, and especially when there is too little water in the body to regulate it. In managing blood pressure, it is important to drink enough water to counteract the extra sodium intake. Still, sodium intake should be restricted to 2,400 mg per day and most of it should come from natural food sources. If you exercise vigorously, you will lose salt through sweating. This allows you to have more sodium without throwing off the balance. In fact, you need to be careful to replace minerals such as sodium and potassium following a workout.

High sodium can throw off the balance of potassium and cause water retention and even kidney failure. The best, most natural way to control it is to drink six to eight glasses of water each day. Eating foods high in potassium will also help regulate sodium and keep blood pressure under control.

Research has also shown that the time of day you consume the most sodium can have as much of an impact on your blood pressure as how much you consume. The research found that women, who ate two-thirds of their daily sodium at dinnertime, had lower blood pressure than those who consumed it at lunchtime.

## KNOCKING HIDDEN SODIUM OUT OF YOUR DIET

The following tips on reducing sodium in your diet are directly from the National Heart, Lung, and Blood Institute's guide for lowering blood pressure.

### Tips to Reduce Salt and Sodium

- Buy fresh, plain frozen, or canned "with no salt added" vegetables.

- Use fresh poultry, fish, and lean meat, rather than canned or processed types.

- Use herbs, spices, and salt-free seasoning blends in cooking and at the table.

- Cook rice, pasta, and hot cereal without salt. Cut back on instant or flavored rice, pasta, and cereal mixes, which usually have added salt.

- Choose "convenience" foods that are low in sodium. Cut back on frozen dinners, pizza, packaged mixes, canned soups or broths, and salad dressings—these often have a lot of sodium.

- Rinse canned foods, such as tuna, to remove some sodium.

- When available, buy low or reduced-sodium or no-salt-added versions of foods.

- Choose ready-to-eat breakfast cereals that are low in sodium.

## WASHING AWAY THE EXCESS: THE ROLE OF WATER

If too much sodium is the "poison," then water may be the "antidote." Anyone who has ever been on a weight-loss diet of any kind has been told by their doctor or dietician that they should have at least eight full glasses of water each day.

Water flushes the body of all kinds of waste and toxins like no other drink can, and it is especially effective in removing excess sodium. You now know that eliminating hidden sodium is a major influence in reducing blood pressure.

Water has no calories or fat. It seems the perfect drink for quenching thirst and replenishing fluid to a dehydrated body. It even works in reducing weight by filling you up so you eat less. It has many health benefits that doctors and scientists have known for years. The bottled water industry has made billions of dollars in educating the rest of us on the importance of drinking water.

Maybe understanding a little about the body will help illustrate the importance of water. The human body is made up mostly of water. It is as vital to life as oxygen. You know what it feels like to be thirsty or dehydrated—you have a dry mouth and maybe even a headache.

What you can't see is what is happening inside the body when it is lacking water. Blood is made up of 85 percent water. When there is not enough water, the blood thickens and its flow can decrease, which, in turn, increases blood pressure.

For the purpose of this book, we are most interested in what water can do to lower blood pressure. However, a lack of water has also been associated with reducing mental sharpness, creating muscle soreness and fatigue, as well as increasing general illness and decreasing the ability to fight disease. Water is life. A lack of water means the end of life—even if it is in the form of a slow deterioration process we don't actually notice.

It is important to begin drinking water *before* you feel thirsty. Once you feel the thirst, you have already become dehydrated to some degree. If you have trouble adding water to your daily routine, try some of the following tips:

- Drink water through a straw.

- Add ice to keep the water cold.

- Use a special cup or bottle just for your water.

- Keep a water bottle by your bedside, in the car, and at your desk, so water is always right in front of you and on your mind.

- Replace other drinks at meals with at least one glass of water.

While there have been concerns raised about water consumption, they do not contradict all of the evidence supporting the need for plenty of water each day.

You should be concerned with the quality of water you drink. Many natural sources of water have trace minerals that are actually harmful. Lead has been found in water, as have high levels of sodium. If you drink water from your tap and it comes from a municipal water supply, it is important to test your water so that you know what is in it. Fortunately, water companies are required to annually publish and distribute to all homes the results of water tests. These will show the mineral content as well as an explanation of what levels are considered safe.

If you have a private well, your water is affected by more than you may think. If your next-door neighbor is dumping motor oil from his last oil change down the drain or into the soil for example, that waste oil is going into your water supply through the ground. You can have your own well tested or visit your local environmental services to get a printout of the ground water makeup for your area.

One sure way to improve the quality of your drinking water is to invest in a high quality filtration system. It may seem like a huge expense, but your health is the ultimate cost. Filtered water can also be tested to show exactly how effective your particular filter is at removing undesirable toxins and minerals.

The emphasis here is to get plenty of water, make sure the water you are drinking is pure, and start lowering your blood pressure by flushing out excess sodium, increasing circulation, and losing weight—all benefits of drinking water.

## WHY ORGANIC?

Organic foods, once only available from the health food store, are now available in more and more supermarkets, thanks to increased demand. Since the public is starting to demand more organically-grown foods, the prices are slowly coming down as supply slowly goes up.

Food labeling laws in the United States make it easy to know that you are really getting organically-grown produce simply by reading the label, or by the fact that they are advertised as "organic."

Just what are organic foods? Organic foods are those without the use of growth-stimulating chemicals (your Miracle Grow type of products) or artificial fertilizers. This is a requirement of using the label "organic." Natural fertilizers are fine, and in fact keep the soils replenished with nutrients that are passed on to the produce. Organic foods must also be grown free of herbicides and insecticides as well.

This designation of organic applies to fresh fruits and vegetables. Adding to their nutritional value is the ripeness. Once a fruit or vegetable passes the peak of ripeness, its natural enzymes can cause them to lose some nutrients. The key here is to eat the fruits and vegetables that are perfectly ripe, not under ripe or past their peak.

Canned fruits and vegetables must be preserved, and thus are not as good for you. The additives of salt for vegetables and sugar for fruits add unnecessary calories. This hidden consumption is a huge factor in raising blood pressure. Because so many processed foods are laced with additives, the average American consumes up to 135 pounds of additives each year—all with little or no nutritional value!

The best way to preserve your fruits and vegetables is to freeze them. You can buy organically-grown vegetables at a good price (or grow your own) during the peak harvesting season and then freeze them. It is important to know that some vegetables need to be blanched in order to keep their fresh taste and texture after freezing. For example, zucchini should be washed, sliced, put into boiling water for one to three minutes, then submerged in cold water to stop the cooking process. The vegetable will still be crunchy and the quick dip in boiling water will not deplete the nutrients.

Most root vegetables—such as carrots, onions, and potatoes—will stay fresh for up to three months if stored in a cool dry place, or even the coldest, humidity-free drawer of the refrigerator. Toward the end of that time, the enzymes will begin to do their job, so it is still best to eat fruits and vegetables in season or pay extra at the market in off-seasons for the imported fruits and vegetables.

Fresh fruits can simply be washed and left to dry before putting them into an airtight container or bag for freezing. It's best to hull fruits like strawberries before freezing. Frozen fruits and vegetables maintain their freshness for three to six months in the freezer or through the off-season in most areas.

## TOP WAYS WE SABOTAGE OUR BLOOD-PRESSURE-LOWERING EFFORTS

Everyone has a vice or two they just can't seem to get out of their life or diet. If yours is alcohol, caffeine, or tobacco and you have high blood pressure, then it's time to find something else to take its place. Fortunately you don't have to completely give up drinking alcohol or coffee, but smoking is another story.

### Alcohol

Alcohol should only be consumed in moderation for several health reasons, but controlling blood pressure is the one we'll focus on here. The American Heart Institute states that more than three drinks a day may increase blood pressure and its related diseases and conditions such as stroke. In addition, alcohol can negate the effect of prescription drugs used to treat hypertension.

The guidelines of acceptable alcohol consumption are clear in the amounts you can drink each day without contributing to hypertension. They are as follows:

**Alcohol Consumption Limits**

|  | Men-Two Drinks | Women-One Drink* |
| --- | --- | --- |
| Examples of what is considered one to two drinks | 24 ounces beer **OR** | 12 ounces beer **OR** |
|  | 10 ounces wine **OR** | 5 ounces wine **OR** |
|  | 2 ounces 100-proof whiskey | 1 ounce 100-proof whiskey |

* This also applies to smaller, lighter-weight men.

## Caffeine

Caffeine has been found to raise blood pressure for short periods of time (and then levels return to normal). So right after that morning cup of coffee you may find your blood pressure readings are high. They will slowly drop as the caffeine leaves your system.

However, if you are one of those people who keeps a constant flow of caffeine going into your system by drinking coffee or caffeinated soft drinks throughout the day, then you are not giving your blood pressure much of a chance to go down.

A study that was presented in 2002 at the annual meeting of the American Society of Hypertension held in New York City indicated caffeine also had an effect on the large arteries in people with hypertension. The author of the study, Charalambos Vlachopoulous, MD, from the Athens Medical School in Greece, stated that caffeine quickly increased the stiffness of the large arteries.

The test Vlachopoulous used gave participants a pill with caffeine equivalent to two to three cups of coffee. It led to an eleven-point jump in systolic blood pressure and an eight-point increase in diastolic blood pressure. This effect lasted for at least three to four hours, peaking after sixty minutes. So, the effect of a morning with two cups of coffee lasts well into the time when you have another cup at the office or at lunch later in the day.

It is important to note that the experts found the study needed further research because that pure form of caffeine the participants received isn't totally realistic. Cream and sugar, for example, can reduce the impact of the caffeine as well as other foods eaten with the coffee. So, before you go cold turkey, you can discuss the amount of coffee you are drinking with your doctor to see if it is negatively impacting your blood pressure.

## Tobacco

Basically, if you have high blood pressure and you smoke, quit! There is no gentle way to put it. Smoking not only contributes to heart disease, stroke, and cancer, but tobacco also increases blood pressure (at least temporarily) and heart rate. It doesn't matter if you smoke it or chew it, the effect is the same.

Smoking tobacco also constricts the arteries, which increases blood pressure. If you smoke and use birth control pills, the effect of tobacco increasing blood pressure is magnified even more.

## CHAPTER SUMMARY

It is probably obvious by now that there are some factors beyond our control in whether or not we will have high blood pressure. Hopefully this chapter emphasized that there is a lot you do have control over, namely your diet and the type of substances you put into your body and what you can avoid to keep your blood pressure down.

Diet is almost always linked with exercise when it comes to maintaining a healthy weight. The same is true when it comes to lowering blood pressure naturally. The next chapter discusses not only exercise, but other forms of movement used to lose weight, strengthen the heart, and reduce stress—all of which help keep blood pressure readings at a healthy level.

# 5

# Where the Rubber Meets the Road: Taking Action to Control and Manage Your Blood Pressure

I can't say enough good things about exercise. There really isn't any type of condition that can't be made at least a little better by improving your overall health and stamina through exercise. Reducing and controlling blood pressure is no exception. The plain and simple truth is that exercise, which leads to a stronger heart and cardiovascular system in general, helps you maintain a healthy weight, which is good for your blood pressure.

## THE BENEFITS OF EXERCISE

The benefits of even moderate exercise can be great. Exercise increases circulation and strengthens muscles, including the heart muscle. It can be beneficial in short, ten-minute stints or longer workouts of forty-five minutes to an hour. You can do as little as twenty minutes, three times per week and see dramatic results in muscle tone, endurance, weight loss, and general well-being.

Unless you become fanatical about exercise, to the point of causing injury to the muscles, there really is no downside to a good workout. So you have nothing to lose (except weight and blood pressure points) and everything to gain from making exercise a part of your everyday life.

Exercise in general needs to become a part of your lifestyle if you are serious about naturally controlling your blood pressure. A good diet and exercise go hand-in-hand, and when the two are ingrained in your mind enough to be a part of each day, you will begin to feel and look better than you ever have. Are there any side effects to exercise? You bet! You will be able to lower your blood pressure without medication by maintaining a healthy weight through proper diet and exercise.

Now, with all we know about the benefits of exercise, one would think that physicians would be advocating exercise for their hypertensive patients as frequently and with as much fanfare as they advise consuming a diet low in sodium. But according to a 2007 study of approximately 17,500 people, all of whom participated in the National Health and Nutrition Examination Survey, two-thirds of the participants were never counseled by their doctors to increase their exercise levels as a way to lower their blood pressure readings (about 4,700 of the participants had hypertension). It's too bad, because among the one-third of patients who did receive counsel from their doctors about increasing their physical activity, 71 percent of them saw a drop in their blood pressure readings. If more people were aware of this, we'd certainly see a significant drop in hypertension rates. As this study's lead researcher pointed out, just a 2 to 3 mmHg drop in the average blood pressure rate would translate to a 25 to 50 percent drop in hypertension diagnoses!

If your blood pressure rates are such that you need to dramatically lower your readings, you can lower your blood pressure significantly by losing just 10 percent of your current body weight. For example, if you are a 5-foot, 10-inch man weighing 200 pounds, and you lose 20 pounds, you will see a drop in blood pressure, even though you may not be at your ideal weight of 165 pounds.

Another benefit to exercise is reduced stress. In the hectic pace of today's world, stress is a reality for most people. Taking time out for yourself and your health should be a top priority.

The sixty-day plan found in Chapter 6 will give you specific exercise plans and a way to track your personal progress. You can use it with the diet plan to lose between eight and sixteen pounds in the sixty days, a loss of one to two pounds per week.

## START DREAMING ABOUT LOWER BLOOD PRESSURE

Sometimes we look for answers to problems by "sleeping on it." This may just be one of the solutions to high blood pressure. Sleep duration has been found to impact the twenty-four-hour per day blood pressure rate, especially for people who get less than six hours per night on average.

Blood pressure does not stay constant throughout the day. As we discussed earlier, consuming a little caffeine in the morning, maybe a cup or two per day of coffee, is okay because it doesn't cause a constant elevation of blood pressure. Blood pressure may rise, but it returns to normal relatively quickly. The opposite is true when it comes to lack of sleep (*good* sleep).

At Columbia University in New York, 4,810 people between the ages of thirty-two and eighty-six were studied during the National Health and Nutrition Examination Survey. Of the participants, 647 had hypertension. The study ruled out causes such as obesity and diabetes, and found that with those between thirty-two and fifty-nine years of age, the common factor for the elevation in their blood pressure was that they were sleeping less than six hours a night. Other studies found that not only did lack of sleep raise the twenty-four-hour blood pressure, but also caused salt retention and elevated sympathetic nervous system activity. All of these contribute to sustained high blood pressure.

The solution to lack of sleep is a simple one for some, more difficult for others. It is easy if you know why you don't get enough sleep. Too much stress and not enough hours in the day to get everything done are among most people's complaints. If you are one of these people, there are some steps you can take to get enough sleep.

1. Don't do your exercising right before bedtime. It can take time to "wind down" from a good workout.

2. Don't eat right before bed. It might make you sleepy, but you will not get the best quality sleep on a very full stomach. Plus it can cause you to gain weight, which increases blood pressure.

3. Plan your time, stick to the plan, and schedule bedtime so that you can get at least seven to nine hours of sleep. If you watch television or read in bed, turn everything off at the scheduled time and don't just fall asleep to the television.

4. If a bed partner's snoring or movement prevents you from getting quality sleep, then you may want separate rooms just for sleeping.

There are sleep disorders and external factors that can prevent you from getting enough sleep, even if you are in bed for eight hours. This can be sleep apnea, where you stop breathing during your sleep, depriving your body of oxygen. It could be insomnia, where you can't get to sleep or stay asleep. These need treatment, probably from a sleep center specializing in sleep disorders.

People who work the night shift also have trouble getting enough quality sleep, even if they are in bed long enough. Make sure the room is completely dark, as it would be at night, and also try to block out phones or other noise that could wake you during the day.

Many studies have linked sleep deprivation to cardiovascular disease. It makes sense that high blood pressure can develop due to continuous sleep deprivation, as the research indicates. Even if there is not an immediate rise in blood pressure after a week of poor sleep, the long-term effects are becoming evident.

## REDUCE YOUR STRESS TO REDUCE YOUR BLOOD PRESSURE

Currently, there is no strong evidence indicating excessive stress causes hypertension. There is, however, proof that stress can temporarily raise blood pressure. By using techniques to reduce stress, you are putting mind over matter in controlling other functions in the body that can contribute to high blood pressure.

One example is that stress reduction is known to help control diet, which we know keeps blood pressure in check. It also just makes you feel better in general.

There are many types of activities that can be used to reduce stress such as:

- Aromatherapy

- Meditation

- Relaxation techniques

- Yoga

- Instant calming sequence

- Biofeedback

Each of these activities can be done at home or in a group setting. They can be done in short sessions or for longer durations. Find what works for you. Find the method that makes you feel less harried. It may be a combination of techniques, depending on a particular day's stress level. Just doing something to take emotional and even physical "time out" can rejuvenate you and get you back into the game, stronger than ever. Let's take a look at each type of stress reducer.

## SMELL YOUR WAY TO LOWER BLOOD PRESSURE

Michael Castleman, author of *The Healing Herbs and Nature's Cures,* talks about aromatherapy as an offshoot of herbal medicine. He explains that the same herbs used by herbalists to heal are also used to create oils and scents that produce similar healing properties.

Valerian root is believed by many herbalists to reduce stress and lower blood pressure. Taken as a tincture, tea, or in pill form, valerian root is used as a natural sedative. Sedation is not really the result you are looking for in reducing stress. So, using the aroma from the valerian root or other mixtures of similar herbs can reduce stress without overmedicating.

Castleman has a stress-reducing recipe in his book for the perfect calming concoction. The ingredients are ones you might already have, or can find at health food and nutrition centers.

- 5 drops of grapefruit oil

- 4 drops cypress

- 2 drops rosemary oil

- 1 teaspoon vegetable oil

- Mix all ingredients together and inhale the aroma or use it to massage the face, neck, shoulders, chest, and back.

## EAT YOUR WAY TO LOWER BLOOD PRESSURE

While it may not do much for your breath, studies show that eating onions can reduce your blood pressure levels. This finding was discovered by researchers from the University in Utah and published in the April 2008 edition of the *Journal of Nutrition*.

The researchers examined the diets and blood pressures of twenty-two patients, all of whom had hypertension, and nineteen pre-hypertensive patients (people with high blood pressure levels, but not high enough to be considered hypertensive). After taking each of their blood pressures at the study's outset, they then gave each of them one of two things: a 730 mg quercetin supplement or a placebo. Quercetin is an antioxidant found in abundant supply in onions. At the study's conclusion, each patient had his or her blood pressure taken again.

Interestingly, the pre-hypertensive patients showed little to no difference in blood pressure levels between the group given a placebo and the group given a supplement. But among the hypertensive group, those given the quercetin supplement had lower blood pressure levels by an average of seven points for the systolic and five points for the diastolic. While these drops may not seem significant, they're significant enough to be the difference between a healthy heart and a heart attack.

Onions not among your favorite vegetables? Well, pick your favorite—just get them into your system! I cannot emphasize enough how important vegetables are to your body, particularly when it comes to those of us with a history of hypertension in our families. According to research performed by Dr. Paul Elliott and colleagues from the Imperial College of London, eating large amounts of vegetables high in protein can work wonders on lowering your blood pressure.

Now, I know what you're thinking: *Protein? In vegetables?* One generally associates protein with meats like beef and poultry. But vegetables are chock-full of protein as well, some more than others.

Before I get to that, though, let's look at the study. Elliott and his colleagues had approximately 4,700 men and women between the ages of forty and fifty-nine participate in their study. Over the course of six weeks, Elliott and his colleagues took each of their blood pressures eight times. Twenty-four hours before each of their blood pressure measurements, Elliott asked that they make a note of everything they ate and drank. Almost uniformly, those who ate large amounts of vegetable protein had progressively lower blood pressure levels compared to those who ate little to no vegetable protein.

What vegetables have the highest levels of protein? The list is long, but a few of them include broccoli, beets, cabbage, kale, artichokes, and cucumbers. Tomatoes are high in vegetable protein as well.

So, really, there's no excuse for not getting some kind of vegetable protein into your diet.

## DRINK YOUR WAY TO LOWER BLOOD PRESSURE

While most of us would rather eat our vegetables than drink them, there's nothing wrong with guzzling them down. In fact, juicing is among the best things you can do to stimulate your energy while at the same time relaxing your heart and keeping your blood pressure at a normal level. One of my favorite concoctions is combining apple, carrots, celery, and beets (The apples give it a fantastic sweetness!).

But, if for some odd reason my mélange doesn't sound appetizing (trust me, you don't know what your missing!), you can create your own delectable delight. In fact, here are some of the high-protein vegetables and fruits that are both delicious and highly "juice-able":

| *Protein Fruits* | *Protein Vegetables* |
| --- | --- |
| Apple | Tomatoes |
| Banana | Spinach |
| Honeydew melon | Zucchini |
| Orange | Cucumber |
| Papaya | Eggplant |
| Pineapple | Green peas |
| Strawberry | Turnip greens |
| Grapes | Beets |

## LISTEN YOUR WAY TO LOWER BLOOD PRESSURE

It's true! Just by listening to music you can lower your blood pressure levels. The trick is in what kind of music it is and for how long you listen to it.

This was discovered after Italian researchers from the University of Florence observed twenty-four participants with mild levels of hypertension. They were instructed to listen to a genre of music—either classical, Celtic, or Indian—for thirty days, thirty minutes per day. They were also instructed to breathe in and out slowly while they were listening.

By the study's conclusion, each of their blood pressure levels had lowered by an average of three points for the systolic and an average of four points for the diastolic. For the sake of comparison, researchers also observed twenty adults for thirty days who were instructed not to listen to the music.

Though the researchers can't say for certain which caused the participants' blood pressures to lower, the music or the slow breathing, they theorized that the combination of slow breathing and relaxing music did the trick. Additional studies, which the chief researcher plans on doing, should further define the causality of music and low blood pressure levels.

## REAPING THE BENEFITS OF MEDITATION

Meditation, in theory, works by removing all thoughts, specifically the stressors in your life, from your mind. This is not an easy task. The way to achieve this is to focus on one word, thought, or even your breath as you clear your mind of everything else.

The natural instinct of a person under stress, which is most of us, is to let your mind wander and focus on your problems. While one school of thought on de-stressing suggests focusing on the problem and doing those things that you have control over, meditation takes the opposite approach.

In the 1970s Dr. Herbert Benson, a Harvard-schooled cardiologist, suggested that meditation was a way to "think" blood pressure lower. He backed his hypothesis through research on monkeys with chronic hypertension.

Benson had hypothesized that the animal kingdom's (humans included) "fight or flight" instinct, which protects us against danger (or stress), greatly contributed to physiological responses of raised heart rate and blood pressure. His findings on meditation showed that by removing the perception of danger—stressors to the animals—from the mind, the coinciding physical reactions were also changed. Heart rate decreased, breathing slowed, and blood pressure lowered.

Meditation takes time. Usually within the first ten minutes, the negative effects are seen. This is mostly because we have been stressed so much and for so long that we just don't know how to relax and get into a truly meditative state.

Here are some techniques to try to shorten the time it takes for the effect of meditation to come into play. It relies on the same type of "mindfulness" as Yoga or Tai Chi. The techniques are summarized as follows from Castleman's book, *Nature's Cures*.

1. Lying on your back, put your arms at your side, palms up, and legs out straight. You can keep your eyes opened or closed.

2. Concentrate on your breathing as each breath flows in and out.

3. Once you start to relax, focus on specific parts of the body. Work from focusing on your toe to your foot. Still be mindful of your breathing. Cas-

tleman suggests imagining you are breathing on the part of the body your attention is on at the moment. Do this for a full minute or two.

4. Follow the same procedure to the next foot and up the body from ankle to knee to thigh to hip.

5. Focus specifically on the face and head with careful attention to the jaw, chin, and lips. He suggests getting very specific with the roof of the mouth, each nostril, and eyelid.

6. You finish by reaching the end of your body, the scalp, and hair. Then you are off the body and "hovering" above yourself with your breath.

This method of meditation is one of many. There are sitting positions with a focus on good posture, but all use the same principles of focusing on breathing and a single thought.

## RELAX FOR LOWER BLOOD PRESSURE: MY FAVORITE TECHNIQUES

There are a number of everyday, simple relaxation techniques that you can use without special training, classes, or taking up a lot of time. Here is the quick list. You can find what works for you. Remember that any relaxation technique is intended to clear the mind of your particular stressors.

- Take a brisk walk. Taking short but brisk ten-minute walks four times a day has been shown to reduce blood pressure for eleven hours. A study published in the September 2006 issue of the *Journal of Hypertension* confirms this.

- Write a to-do list so you can stop worrying about all that you need to accomplish.

- Stretch. Sounds simple, but stretching the neck, arms, and back can relieve the pressure there and quickly rejuvenate your body.

- Take action. Do what you can about the things over which you have control. Delegate what you can't or don't want to handle.

## THE TRUTH ABOUT YOGA AND BLOOD PRESSURE

Yoga works like meditation and exercise in encouraging deep breathing and flexibility. A study conducted in 1993 in India analyzed the effects of yoga on a group of people who were generally physically active and in good health—physical education teachers. The forty participants had their basic vital statistics measured, including blood pressure.

The results were somewhat surprising for such a fit group of people—they found blood pressure was lowered after just three months of training. Also, improvement was realized in lung function, heart and breathing rates, and even hand steadiness.

To practice yoga in the most beneficial way, you probably need to be led by a professional. If you have the luxury of a private instructor, you can improve quickly (depending on how much time you can devote to it).

Most people will find that a group class at a local YMCA or gym is more realistic than private sessions. You can also benefit from using a videotape at home. There are several types of American and Chinese yoga programs at various levels, so you can increase your performance and the benefits when you are ready.

## THE SUREFIRE INSTANT CALMING SEQUENCE

There may be days or times when it is unrealistic to light a candle and take a bubble bath to relax you. You may be on the road for work and unable to attend your yoga class, for example. For occasions such as these, there is a six-step process called the Instant Calming Sequence, developed by Dr. Robert Cooper, Ph.D., president of the Institute of Health and Fitness Excellence in Minnesota. His quick-fix relaxation plan can be done anywhere, anytime you feel your stress level rising out of control.

Here is how it works:

- Step 1: Practice uninterrupted breathing. Breathe smoothly, deeply, and evenly, focusing on each breath.

- Step 2: Put on a positive face. You smile when you are happy and Dr. Cooper believes it works both ways. When you smile, you actually make yourself feel happy.

- Step 3: Balance your posture. Dr. Cooper has found that posture works like smiling. When you sit up straight, you feel better. People who are stressed tend to hunch with the weight of their troubles. Remove the slouch and you work toward removing the troubles causing it.

- Step 4: Bathe in a wave of relaxation. Visualize that you are literally being washed with a wave from a waterfall that is cleansing away the stress-causing situation.

- Step 5: Acknowledge reality. Dr. Cooper counsels that you should face your stressor head on. Denial is a temporary, ineffective way of reducing stress. Use positive thoughts and words to reassure yourself that this is reality and that you can handle it.

- Step 6: Reassert Control: Focus on the controllable aspects of the stressful situation and do what you can. Again, don't deny the problem, but face it realistically.

## BIOFEEDBACK FOR LOWER BLOOD PRESSURE

Biofeedback has been determined by many medical professionals as a viable way to reduce blood pressure in some people. It is a relaxation technique that goes one step beyond others such as yoga or meditation in that it requires monitoring and measuring the results of learned relaxation methods. That way you can determine how well they are working and eventually be able to apply them daily or as needed without monitoring.

In general, most involuntary bodily functions cannot be controlled with the mind. The premise behind biofeedback is that if you can see, in measurable output, the results of willing yourself to relax mentally, then you can use these techniques anytime and anywhere. Understanding how the body responds to thoughts is what makes biofeedback a good tool in lowering blood pressure. However, it will not take the place of the more physical or tangible methods of a good diet, proper weight maintenance, and challenging exercise.

Studies have shown that relaxing and reducing mental stress causes the arteries to relax and lowers blood pressure. When we have stress, the blood vessels constrict, especially in the extremities, which makes them colder. With biofeedback, the patient can learn to recognize when stress is restricting blood flow to the extremities and warm up the fingers and toes in order to dilate the blood vessels and lower blood pressure.

There are two important factors to consider with biofeedback. The first is that it requires a professional to administer the process. Electrodes are painlessly attached to the body in several locations to measure brain activity, body temperature, heart rate, and, with hypertension patients, blood pressure. Other involuntary bodily responses can be measured, but these are the most common. A trained and licensed therapist can properly measure the physiological responses.

However, it requires another step, which is learning how to change the responses. The ability to mentally control a response based on the biofeedback reading in a clinical setting can be implemented outside of that clinical setting.

The second major consideration with biofeedback is that it cannot be used initially with essential hypertension. Proper medical care should be used to control the immediate blood pressure issue. For pre-hypertensive people, biofeedback can be used early on. If the therapy is effective based on consistent monitoring of blood pressure, great! If not, further action should be taken. This would include losing weight if necessary, changing eating habits, increasing exercise, etc.

Most medical professionals agree that biofeedback can't hurt. It is one more way to actively change your thinking and lifestyle and control blood pressure without the use of medication. You can use the information to employ stress reduction techniques that work for you by examining how your blood pressure responds based on the biofeedback.

## HAPPINESS IS LOWER BLOOD PRESSURE

It may sound a little too simple, but being happy has been proven to keep a heart healthy. A condition known as metabolic syndrome is where other health conditions such as high blood pressure, high blood sugar, and elevated cholesterol, along with carrying excessive fat in the abdominal area, are found together. These all can lead to heart disease and/or stroke.

A twelve-year study of more than 400 women concluded that those who were happy in their marriages and happy in general were less likely to develop metabolic syndrome. Likewise, happy single women had the same lower occurrences as the happily married women.

The study went on to control factors that may have contributed to the results, such as age, race, and lifestyle choices, including exercise levels and whether or not the women smoked. When those factors were controlled, the results were the same. Happier women were less likely to develop the pre-cursors to heart disease, including high blood pressure.

Being happy may be as much a state of mind and attitude as controlling stress willfully. In fact, a psychologist referring to this study believes it is possible that the stress caused by an unhappy marriage can cause elevated blood pressure readings. Choosing to be happy and positive, and reducing the stressors you can control, will work with diet and exercise to maintain healthy blood pressure readings.

## MAPPING OUT YOUR OWN EXERCISE PLAN

### Talk to Your Doctor

To find out what kind of exercise and stress-reducing plans will work for you in your quest to get healthier and lower your blood pressure, you need to talk to your doctor.

Everyone's starting point will be different. An exercise plan for someone fifty pounds overweight will be different from a plan for someone who only needs to drop ten pounds. Also, your doctor will be able to suggest what level of activity is appropriate and safe for your overall health.

### *Evaluate Your Interests and Capabilities*

Beyond the physical factors in setting up your own exercise plan, there are emotional considerations. No exercise plan will work if you don't stick with it because you think it is too difficult or boring.

The first step, then, after talking to your doctor, is to evaluate your interests. If the thought of dancing around an aerobics class with a bunch of other people makes you want to run the other way, then consider something you can do outdoors or on your own. Remember, even little changes in movement can have big results.

If you are fifty and have never been running, then jogging and preparing for a marathon may not be the best choice for you. It certainly is an attainable goal if that is what really interests you, but you would be better served by starting a walking or swimming routine and working your way up to longer walks, jogs, and then all-out marathons.

There are cardiovascular benefits to other forms of exercise that are disguised as fun. Play soccer in the yard with your children, or walk along behind them as they learn to ride their bikes. Throw a ball to the dog, and try to get it back again. Before you know it you will have raised your heart rate for the recommended twenty-minute stint. You don't have to get into special clothes, drive some place, and take up hours of your time to get moving! Raking leaves, shoveling snow, cleaning the house, and going out dancing for the night can all be turned into workouts.

## FITTING EXERCISE INTO YOUR EVERYDAY LIFE

You need to make exercise a priority if it is going to help you. You could think about it like this: If you don't make time for exercise now, you will have to make time for the heart disease that will eventually come from untreated hypertension.

Here are some of the tried-and-true methods to getting involved in more physical activity without having to set aside a big chunk of time:

- Take the stairs instead of the elevator whenever possible.

- Park at the far end of the parking lot instead of finding the closest space to the building.

- Get a dog or find another friend who would like to take walks with you. A dog is a great motivator. If you don't walk him, you'll both pay the price!

- Turn off the power propel on your lawn mower and use your own power to push.

- If you are a couch potato, then move to the floor and do leg lift exercises, or work with hand weights as you watch the news.

## CHAPTER SUMMARY

You need to move to get your heart healthy and lower your blood pressure. It is never too late to start getting more exercise into your everyday life. Following the advice of your doctor, start something that you can live with day after day, week after week, and year after year.

The benefits of exercise are countless. Not only will you lose weight and reduce stress, which in turn will lower blood pressure, but you will also have greater vitality in every other part of your life. The physical benefits will be complemented by the mental rewards of a clearer mind and, for most people, a better outlook on life that results from feeling your best.

# 6

# The Sixty-Day Plan

Now that you have an understanding of what you are able to do on your own to lower your blood pressure naturally, it is time to put that knowledge into action. The sixty-day plan is intended to be the first sixty-days in a lifelong pattern of good eating and exercise habits.

This sixty-day plan is not a quick-fix solution. It is not a fad diet plan that helps you lose the first ten percent of your weight loss goal and then allows you to go back to old habits. The harm of untreated high blood pressure takes years to realize. So it makes sense that it takes years of healthy blood pressure to reap the rewards. The results after sixty days will be enough for you to make this type of behavior a lifelong routine.

During the sixty days, you will probably lose a significant amount of weight. You will see a difference in your energy level. You will see a positive change in your blood pressure readings and hopefully make the transition from relying on medicine to a more natural form of treating your high blood pressure.

This sixty-day plan is like other habit-changing programs in that you will set goals, and then focus on one goal at a time for about a week. It involves replacing old habits with new ones. It is difficult to remove a familiar, comfortable habit—especially the bad ones—if you don't replace it with something else.

Let's say, for example, that you love to eat a bowl of ice cream each night before bed. It's your way of rewarding yourself for all the hard work you've done, and it's a quiet, relaxing experience for you to eat a couple of scoops in front of the television at night.

When you set a goal of limiting ice cream consumption to one day a week, you need to replace the other six times in the week with something else. Remember, this is to be a lifetime change, so unless you plan to never eat ice cream again, going to one serving per week is good. You could indulge in some other treat that is healthier than ice cream.

Once you have made the change a part of your new way of doing things, you will move on to the next change while maintaining the first.

As the changes add up, you will discover at the end of sixty-days that you have both removed old habits that contributed to high blood pressure and added new measures to lower your blood pressure and maintain a healthy lifestyle.

*Week 1: Make an appointment with your doctor to discuss plans and determine which supplements will benefit you most. Create reasonable diet and exercise plans.*

## ADDING SUPPLEMENTS

Part of the plan to lower blood pressure naturally is to add supplements known to do the job. There is a step-by-step method, set out by the experts at WholeHealthmd.com, to adding supplements and monitoring their effectiveness. Ideally, careful food choices would allow you to get all of the minerals without too many calories, but sometimes a supplement helps make up for shortages in the diet.

The recommended way of adding supplements is to start with calcium and magnesium. Add 1,000 mg of calcium and 500 mg magnesium to your diet for one month. After taking these supplements for four weeks, see if your blood pressure lowers. If not, try adding up to 1,000 mg more of potassium through dietary changes, such as having a banana and yogurt between meals. No one should take a potassium supplement without consulting their doctor, *especially* if they have kidney problems. If you do not see positive results with this and your other lifestyle changes of diet, exercise, limited alcohol and tobacco use, then try taking vitamin C with hawthorn or coenzyme Q10. You can also add two extra servings of fish each week or a fish oil supplement.

It may be your diet changes alone add enough of the vitamins and minerals you need, but the supplements ensure you are getting the blood-pressure-lowering benefits of these nutrients. Once you know you are getting the needed vitamins and minerals from your diet, you can lower the amounts of the supplements.

## Recommended Supplements

If, by chance, you're not getting the kind of supplementation you need from food sources to lower your blood pressure, then you definitely want to stick with supplements. Here are some of the best supplements to take for lowering blood pressure levels; they're also ones I use regularly and highly recommend:

### Coenzyme Q10

As previously mentioned, coenzyme Q10 is a great supplement to take, particularly if you want to promote healthy cardiac function. But as you might imagine, there are several coenzyme Q10 products to choose from (*several* is an understatement). One of my favorites is made by Jarrow Formulas. It's called QH-absorb and comes in a variety of dosages, from 30 mg up to 200 mg.

### Garlic

If it didn't seep through the body's pores, unleashing a rather objectionable odor, garlic would be a significant part of my daily diet. However, thanks to garlic supplements, I can get the benefits garlic has on cardiovascular function, minus its sinful scent.

My favorite garlic supplement is made by Wakunaga of America and is called Kyolic. You should have no problem finding Kyolic at General Nutrition Center (GNC) and Vitamin Shoppe stores.

In your travels for these and other supplements, you'll see for yourself the array of choices. Nature's Way is a well known company that you can always count on for quality and reliability. Whether you're looking for homeopathic remedies, herbs, essential fatty acids, or minerals, you can rest assured Nature's Way produces a quality product that will suit your needs.

## Menu Planning

The first week of your sixty-day plan needs to include careful menu planning. After a few weeks, you will have the habits formed to make good choices at the grocery store, restaurants, and at home without having to think so much about each choice.

By planning your menu ahead of time, you accomplish two things: a more focused shopping trip with good choices and the elimination of the need to rethink every choice each day. The objective here is to make a lifestyle change that doesn't control your life, but where *you* have control over your lifestyle.

Use the following menu planning chart to plan your menu. Choose fresh, unprocessed foods as much as possible. Then use the shopping list to make sure you have everything you need.

## Exercise Plan

By now you should know the importance of adding exercise to your plan. It will strengthen your muscles including the heart, and help in your weight loss goals. Now is the time to determine what exercise you will enjoy enough to stick with it, and create some variety to your plan for added interest. Also, here you will map out time for that exercise.

Just like everything else in your hectic life, you can and must schedule exercise. Use your day planner, calendar, or handheld electronic organizer to schedule your exercise as you would all other important appointments.

Complete the following questionnaire to help create an exercise plan. Check off your answers.

1. What time of day do you like to exercise most?

❑ First thing in the morning

❑ Mid-day

❑ After work

❑ After dinner/late evening

## Weekly Menu Planner

| Day | 1 | 2 | 3 | 4 | 5 | 6 | 7 |
|-----|---|---|---|---|---|---|---|
| Breakfast | | | | | | | |
| Lunch | | | | | | | |
| Dinner | | | | | | | |
| Snacks | | | | | | | |

# Shopping List

| Fruits/Vegetables | Dairy | Fish/Meat/Poultry | Grains | Other |
|---|---|---|---|---|
|  |  |  |  |  |
|  |  |  |  |  |
|  |  |  |  |  |
|  |  |  |  |  |
|  |  |  |  |  |
|  |  |  |  |  |
|  |  |  |  |  |
|  |  |  |  |  |
|  |  |  |  |  |
|  |  |  |  |  |
|  |  |  |  |  |
|  |  |  |  |  |
|  |  |  |  |  |
|  |  |  |  |  |
|  |  |  |  |  |

2. What days of the week will you exercise? (Check all that apply.)

❑  Sunday

❑  Monday

❑  Tuesday

❑  Wednesday

❑  Thursday

❑  Friday

❑  Saturday

3. Do you like to exercise alone or with a friend?

❑  Alone

❑  With a Friend

4. Does your exercise plan require any special equipment?

❑  Yes

❑  No

5. Has your exercise plan been approved by your doctor?

❑  Yes

❑  No

6. Write down your exercise goals. For example: distance to walk/run, time to walk/run, amount of weight to lift, number of repetitions for exercise.

### Weeks 2 through 8: Set goals for behavior changes.

The first week of the plan was about getting organized and ready to make a lifelong change. Starting with the second week and each week thereafter, you will set a goal to change a habit or behavior from one that is detrimental to your blood pressure to one that will make you healthier. You will focus only on this goal for the week. By the next week it will be a part of your routine and eventually become a lasting change. Then you can start the new week focusing on one more behavioral change.

**Exercise Plan**

| Type of exercise | Week #(1–8) | Goal |
|---|---|---|
| Example: Walking | Week 1 | 20 min each day/3 days |
| | | |
| | | |
| | | |
| | | |
| | | |
| | | |
| | | |
| | | |
| | | |

For any goal to be accomplished, it must be clear and specific. The actions toward achieving the goal must be something you can control. Here are some examples:

- Drink eight glasses of water each day

- Do not eat after 8 p.m.

- Meditate to reduce stress each evening

- Cut three cigarettes from daily total

- Cut one alcoholic beverage from daily total

- Eat two fruit servings

- Count to ten and take deep breaths before yelling

- Cut out two cups of coffee from daily total

- Cut table salt from cooking and meals; replace with other sodium-free seasonings

Focusing on these weekly changes, you will determine which habits you have that are hurting your blood pressure. These will be individual goals and changes based on your current weak areas. Some people may not smoke, so that won't be an issue. They may, however, eat a lot of pre-packaged foods and add table salt to everything; they will need to find a way to cut down on their sodium consumption.

## KEEPING TRACK

The journal page should be copied for each of the sixty days. Here you will record your goals and accomplishments, including your feelings about how well you think you did.

## Sixty-Day Journal
## for Lowering Blood Pressure Naturally

Day: _____ Date: _____ Blood Pressure Reading: _____

Weight: _____

Weekly Goal Focus: _____

Exercise Accomplished: _____

_____

### *Food Journal:*

Breakfast: _____

Lunch: _____

Dinner: _____

Snacks: _____

Water: _____ Alcohol: _____ Tobacco: _____

Thoughts/Feelings/Observations: _____

_____

_____

## The Sixty-Day Plan Calendar

The following calendar summarizes how you can make changes each day and week. It gives you a daily task that is manageable and can fit into anyone's daily routine. You can look ahead, but as you start the plan, you can choose to focus only on that day's task and the goal or objective for the week ahead. It is intended to help you stay focused on all the little changes that add up to bigger results. Use the calendar with the forms and charts for setting your own goals, accomplishing each task, and measuring the results.

## A LIFELONG CHANGE

You have done it! You've committed yourself to a healthier way of managing your blood pressure through good nutrition, exercise, and a strong mental outlook. After sixty days you will be able to see the results. You will feel it in looser clothing, your renewed sense of energy, and your increased physical and mental strength. You will see it in cold, hard numbers. Lower numbers will appear on the scale, and most importantly, in your daily or weekly blood pressure readings.

The sixty days are the pattern for a lifelong way of managing stress and controlling that which only you can control—what goes into your body and the output you give through exercise. Your habits are reformed by the end of sixty days. Continue with the changes, and add new ones if you still have areas where you need to make changes in lifestyle in order to live a prescription-free life of healthy blood pressure.

This is the conclusion of the sixty-day plan, but the beginning of the rest of your life. By making the changes that lower your blood pressure, it will be a longer, healthier life. It is within your power and control to lower your blood pressure and live life to the fullest.

Wishing You the Very Best of Health,

*Frank Mangano*

Frank Mangano
Consumer Health Advocate
www.NaturalHealthOnTheWeb.com
F.Mangano@verizon.net

**Calendar for Days 1 through 30**

| Day 1 | Day 2 | Day 3 | Day 4 | Day 5 | Day 6 | Day 7 |
|---|---|---|---|---|---|---|
| Call doctor to make appointment to discuss plans and get approval. Take brisk walk. | Fill out weekly menu. Buy calcium, magnesium, and potassium if advised by your doctor. | Write out food shopping list. Take brisk walk. | Go to grocery store. Use meditation technique to relax after work. | Doctor's appointment. Start taking 1000 mg calcium (with approval) | Add 500 mg magnesium daily. Exercise for thirty minutes. | Add a banana or other potassium-rich food to your diet. Record weight. |
| This week: Set up exercise plan to include three thirty-minute workouts each day. Take blood pressure reading at the same time each day, and record on journal page. | | | | | | |
| Day 8 | Day 9 | Day 10 | Day 11 | Day 12 | Day 13 | Day 14 |
| Begin second weekly habit change. Exercise. | Replace one cup of today's coffee with a tall glass of ice water with lemon. | Write in journal your feelings about your plan so far. Exercise. | Do grocery shopping for next seven days. | Exercise five minutes longer than your last workout. | Call a friend for support and tell them about your new habits. | Begin your cardio workout with a fifteen-minute meditation session. Record weight |
| This week: Set weekly goal for behavior change. Exercise three times. Write in journal each day. | | | | | | |
| Day 15 | Day 16 | Day 17 | Day 18 | Day 19 | Day 20 | Day 21 |
| Add new type of exercise to your routine. | Buy notebook for writing down thoughts, items to do that are stressing you out. | Add weight to your arms as you walk. | Do grocery shopping for next seven days. | Exercise ten minutes longer than your last workout. | Concentrate on keeping your posture straighter as you sit and stand. | Record weight in journal. |
| This week: Set weekly goal for behavior change. Exercise four times. Write in journal each day. | | | | | | |
| Day 22 | Day 23 | Day 24 | Day 25 | Day 26 | Day 27 | Day 28 |
| Add new type of exercise to your routine. | Go to meals.com and try a new low-fat, high-fiber recipe. | Try Instant Calming Sequence (p. 63). | Do grocery shopping for next seven days. | Practice deep breathing when under stress. | Buy new item of clothing in a smaller size. (Your weight loss will be four to ten pounds!) | Record weight in journal. |
| This week: Set weekly goal for behavior change. Exercise four times. Write in journal each day. | | | | | | |
| Day 29 | Day 30 | | | | | |
| Add new type of exercise to your routine. | Evaluate supplements, discuss with your doctor. Make any necessary changes. | | | | | |

**Calendar for Days 31 through 60**

| | | | | | | |
|---|---|---|---|---|---|---|
| Day 31 Add new type of exercise to your routine. | Day 32 Practice stretching before you get out of bed. | Day 33 Do online search for "heart-healthy foods" to add to your menu plan. | Day 34 Do grocery shopping for next seven days. | Day 35 De-stress by cleaning out your wallet. | Day 36 Exercise fifteen minutes longer than you did your last workout. | Day 37 Record weight in journal. |
| This week: Set weekly goal for behavior change. Exercise five times. Write in journal each day. | | | | | | |
| Day 38 Add new type of exercise to your routine. | Day 39 Try a new fish recipe for dinner. | Day 40 Start hobby you have been putting off. | Day 41 Do grocery shopping for next seven days. | Day 42 Take thirty minutes to do something nice for yourself. | Day 43 De-stress by organizing your top desk drawer. | Day 44 Record weight in journal. |
| This week: Set weekly goal for behavior change. Exercise five times. Write in journal each day. | | | | | | |
| Day 45 Add new type of exercise to your routine. | Day 46 Find three dinner recipes that include more fresh garlic and less salt to add to your diet. | Day 47 Go online and find new way to add interest to a walking workout. | Day 48 Do grocery shopping for next seven days. | Day 49 De-stress by completing unfinished project around the house. | Day 50 Visit a farmers' market for fresh fruits and vegetables. | Day 51 Record weight in journal. |
| This week: Set weekly goal for behavior change. Exercise five times. Write in journal each day. | | | | | | |
| Day 52 Add new type of exercise to your routine. | Day 53 De-stress by cleaning out one file drawer at home or work. | Day 54 Try new kind of vegetable. | Day 55 Do grocery shopping for next seven days. | Day 56 Play game of one-on-one driveway basketball | Day 57 Treat yourself to a professional massage. | Day 58 Record weight in journal. |
| This week: Set weekly goal for behavior change. Exercise five times. Write in journal each day. | | | | | | |
| Day 59 Determine any additional habits you want to change. Write them down. | Day 60 Evaluate results over the last fifty-nine days. Plan for the next thirty days. | | | | | |

# References

## BOOKS

*Archives of Internal Medicine,* May 9, 2005. (Happiness and heart health study)

Balch, Phyllis A., *Prescription For Nutritional Healing,* third edition, CNC, Avery, 2000.

Castleman, Michael, *Nature's Cures,* Rodale Press, Inc., 1996.

Goldbeck, Mikki and David, *The Dieter's Companion—A Guide to Nutritional Self-Sufficiency,* McGraw-Hill, 1977.

*Mann, S.J., M.D., Healing Hypertension: Uncovering the Secret Power of Your Hidden Emotions,* John Wiley and Sons, 1999.

Null, Gary, Ph.D, *The Complete Encyclopedia Of Natural Healing,* Kensington, 1998.

Pelletier, Kenneth R., MD, *Best Alternative Medicine,* Simon & Schuster, 2000.

Rowan, R., M.D., et al, *Control High Blood Pressure Without Drugs,* Simon & Schuster, 2001.

Whitaker, J., M.D., *Reversing Hypertension: A Vital New Program to Prevent, Treat, and Reduce High Blood Pressure,* Warner Books, 2000.

## ONLINE RESOURCES

American Heart Association Online Resources:
www.americanheart.org
Bison Basics:
www.bisonbasics.com/nutrition/nutrition.html
Health Journal:
www.bodyandfitness.com/Information/Health/bloodpressure.htm.
Herbs 200 Resources:
www.herbs2000.com/disorders/high_blood.htm
Johns Hopkins Medical Library News Releases:
www.hopkinsmedicine.org/press
Mayo Clinic:
www.mayoclinic.com/health/alpha-blockers/hi00055
MedicWeb Resources:
hypertension.medicweb.org/alternative/blood_pressure_and_herbs.php
Medline Plus Drug Information:
www.nlm.nih.gov
Mercola Resources:
www.mercola.com
National Heart, Lung, and Blood Institute:
www.nhlbi.nih.gov.
National Library of Medicine Journals Database:
www.ncbi.hih.gov.
Natural News Resources:
www.naturalnews.com/022779.html, www.naturalnews.com/021427.html,
www.naturalnews.com/020173.html, www.naturalnews.com/022987.html
www.naturalnews.com/025189.html
New York Times:
www.nytimes.com/2008/12/30/science/30baby.html
Reuters:
www.reuters.com/article/healthNews/idUSLAU48158320070725
Science Daily:
www.sciencedaily.com/releases/2008/12/081229200733.htm
www.sciencedaily.com/releases/2008/11/081109074611.htm
Science Links Japan:
sciencelinks.jp/j-east/article/200123/000020012301A0773165.php
Supplement Resources:
www.jarrow.com/ and www.naturesway.com/
U.S. News & World Report:
health.usnews.com/articles/health/healthday/2008/08/14/exercise-reduces-blood-
pressure.html
WebMD Health Guide:
www.webmd.com/hw/health_guide and www.webmd.com/hypertension-high-blood-
pressure/news/20080514/relax-to-music-ease-blood-pressure
www.webmd.com/hypertension-high-blood-pressure/tc/high-blood-pressure-hypertension-
medications
Whole Health MD:
www.wholehealthmd.com.
Vegetable Resources:
www.happycow.net/vegetarian_protein.html

# About Frank Mangano

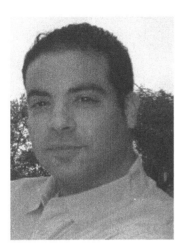

In today's world it seems as though everyone is preoccupied with living a healthier lifestyle. With this in mind, the pharmaceutical companies and prescription drug manufacturers find themselves in a position of power that was never even conceivable until now.

There are, however, a handful of driven researchers putting forth numerous efforts to seek concepts and solutions to health dilemmas minus the interest in the all-mighty dollar sign.

Frank Mangano is a consumer health advocate and natural health writer who has authored and published numerous reports and a considerable amount of articles pertaining to natural health. He teaches you how to dramatically improve your health naturally, without expensive and potentially dangerous prescription drugs.

The hard work and persistence that Frank has invested in is reflected through his writings, which are available at http://www.NaturalHealthOnTheWeb.com .